Extemporaneous Formulations for Pediatric, Geriatric, and Special Needs Patients

second edition

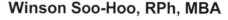

Rita K. Jew, PharmD, FASHP
Executive Director
Department of Pharmacy and Clinical Nutrition Services
Children's Hospital of Orange County
Orange County, California

Winson Soo-Hoo, RPh, MBA
Director
Department of Pharmacy Services
The Children's Hospital of Philadelphia
Philadelphia, Pennsylvania

Sarah C. Erush, PharmD, BCPS
Clinical Manager
Department of Pharmacy Services
The Children's Hospital of Philadelphia
Philadelphia, Pennsylvania

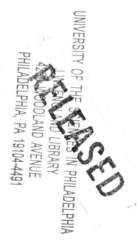

American Society of Health–System Pharmacists®
Bethesda, Maryland

Any correspondence regarding this publication should be sent to the publisher, American Society of Health-System Pharmacists, 7272 Wisconsin Avenue, Bethesda, MD 20814, attention: Special Publishing.

The information presented herein reflects the opinions of the contributors and advisors. It should not be interpreted as an official policy of ASHP or as an endorsement of any product.

Because of ongoing research and improvements in technology, the information and its applications contained in this text are constantly evolving and are subject to the professional judgment and interpretation of the practitioner due to the uniqueness of a clinical situation. The editors, contributors, and ASHP have made reasonable efforts to ensure the accuracy and appropriateness of the information presented in this document. However, any user of this information is advised that the editors, contributors, advisors, and ASHP are not responsible for the continued currency of the information, for any errors or omissions, and/or for any consequences arising from the use of the information in the document in any and all practice settings. Any reader of this document is cautioned that ASHP makes no representation, guarantee, or warranty, express or implied, as to the accuracy and appropriateness of the information contained in this document and specifically disclaims any liability to any party for the accuracy and/or completeness of the material or for any damages arising out of the use or non-use of any of the information contained in this document.

Director, Special Publishing: Jack Bruggeman

Acquisitions Editor: Jack Bruggeman

Senior Editorial Project Manager: Dana Battaglia

Production Editor: Kristin Eckles

Cover: Carol Barrer

Page Design and Composition: David Wade

ISBN: 978-1-58528-245-6

Table of Contents

Part I: Elixir/Solution/Suspension/Syrup

Part II: Ointment/Ophthalmic Solution

Part III: Commercially Available Products

Use extemporaneously prepared formulation only when commercial product is unavailable or a more dilute or more concentrated product is desired.

Appendices

Preface to the First Edition

The lack of commercially available oral liquid formulations poses a frequent challenge in providing medications to pediatric patients, geriatric patients, patients with feeding tubes, and patients who cannot swallow solid dosage forms. Pharmacists are often required to prepare extemporaneous formulations of oral solutions and suspensions to meet the needs of these patients. As highlighted by a survey performed by Crawford and colleagues,[1] pharmacists are performing a broad range of extemporaneous compounding activities from preparing oral solutions and suspensions to compounding ophthalmic solutions and suppositories. It is also apparent from the respondents of the survey that there is a need for stability and other information on extemporaneous drug formulations.

The American Society of Health-System Pharmacists (ASHP, formerly American Society of Hospital Pharmacists) Special Interest Group on Pediatric Pharmacy Practice formed a subcommittee in 1977 to examine the issue of extemporaneously prepared formulations. The report of the Subcommittee on Pediatric Extemporaneous Formulations was published in 1979. Since that time, there have been several publications on extemporaneous formulations, but most of them have been lacking in stability data.

At The Children's Hospital of Philadelphia, an examination of our extemporaneous formulations in 1996 showed that many of them were based on older references, such as the ASHP or Canadian Extemporaneous Formulations Handbook, where stability data were lacking. In addition, some key ingredients, such as Cologel, were no longer commercially available. Therefore, in 1997, the Department of Pharmacy Services initiated a project to research all extemporaneous formulations on file. Old references were reviewed and a comprehensive literature search was performed to identify new information and formulations. In addition, pharmaceutical manufacturers were contacted when no information was readily available in the literature. This compilation was completed after one year and the new formulations were maintained in an Access database. The information was updated in 2002. Because we share this information with chain, community, and hospital pharmacies on a regular basis, we decided to partner with ASHP to publish this information so that it can be readily available to the pharmacy community.

This book only contains formulations that have published and documented stability data. We decided to list the various published formulations of each medication so that readers can choose the most appropriate formulation of each medication for their patients. Only a few ophthalmic preparations are included because of the lack of published data. Also included in this compilation are formulations that were developed before the availability of the commercially manufactured products. These formulations are handy during drug shortages, such as those for famotidine and mycophenolate suspensions. To comply with FDA regulations, these formulations should only be used when the commercially available products are unavailable or when the commercially available concentration is not desirable for the specific patient or patient population.

Although this book was created with pediatric patients in mind, it is intended to serve as a resource for all pharmacies—especially those with a large geriatric population. It will also be of value to community pharmacies that routinely compound prescriptions extemporaneously for pediatric or geriatric patients and pharmacies that service long-term care institutions. We hope that this handbook will become as valuable a resource to you as it has been for us.

Reference

Crawford SY, Dombrowski SR. Extemporaneous compounding activities and the associated informational needs of pharmacists. *Am J Hosp Pharm*. 1991;48:1205–10.

Preface to the Second Edition

It has been seven years since the publication of *Extemporaneous Formulations*. Despite the FDA Best Pharmaceuticals for Children's Act of 2002 that offers incentive to pharmaceutical manufacturers for pediatric research, a gap still exists in pharmaceuticals with appropriate pediatric formulations. Pharmacists continue to bridge this gap by preparing extemporaneous formulations. With the new edition of this book, we performed another comprehensive literature search to identify new drugs with extemporaneous formulations and new formulations of drugs that are in the first edition of the book. As with the previous edition, only formulations that have published and documented stability data are included. We continue to provide multiple published formulations of medications with the same concentration as well as formulations with various concentrations so that readers can choose the most appropriate formulation for their patients. However, we have excluded formulations that are impractical to make (mainly from old references from Europe) and concentrations that are of no practical value (e.g., midazolam 0.035 mg/ml) in the event that there are numerous formulations with various concentrations published in the literature. This exercise has resulted in the expansion of formulations from 107 to 160. In this edition, we have also included study container type when the information is available in the published article. It is probably appropriate to store most formulations in a plastic container. However, when the stability study is performed in a glass container, it is best to store the formulation in a glass container until additional data is available. We continue to recommend storing the extemporaneously compounded formulations in a light-resistant container. However, we specify "protect form light" in a few formulations where the compound is light sensitive in order to stress the importance of this storage condition.

Despite the fact that we have spent endless hours compiling published formulations in the second edition of *Extemporaneous Formulations,* our work cannot be compared to the tireless work of individuals such as Drs Loyd Allen, Cary Johnson, and Milap Nahata to name a few, who continue to conduct stability studies of extemporaneous formulations and contribute to the literature to benefit the patients we take care of. We hope *Extemporaneous Formulations* will help improve and optimize the care of your patients as much as it has for ours.

Introduction

Legal Considerations

Before a pharmacist engages in extemporaneous compounding activities, it is important to understand the legal implications. Extemporaneous formulations compounded by pharmacists for individual patients are entitled to exemptions from the three provisions (adulteration, misbranding, and new drug provisions) of the Food and Drug Modernization Act. To qualify for these statutory exemptions, pharmacists must not engage in the following activities per the FDA compliance policy guide 460.200[1]:

- Compounding of drugs in anticipation of receiving prescriptions, except in very limited quantities in relation to the amounts of drugs compounded after receiving valid prescriptions;
- Compounding drugs that were withdrawn or removed from the market for safety reasons (Appendix A of reference 1);
- Compounding finished drugs from bulk active ingredients that are not components of FDA-approved drugs without an FDA-sanctioned investigational new drug application;
- Receiving, storing, or using drug substances without first obtaining written assurance from the supplier that each lot of the drug substance was made in an FDA-registered facility;
- Receiving, storing, or using drug components not guaranteed or otherwise determined to meet official compendia requirements;
- Using commercial-scale manufacturing or testing equipment for compounding drug products;
- Compounding drugs for third parties who resell to individual patients or offering compounded drug products at wholesale price to other state licensed persons or commercial entities for resale;
- Compounding drug products that are commercially available in the marketplace or that are essentially copies of commercially available FDA-approved drug products. In certain circumstances, it may be appropriate for a pharmacist to compound a small quantity of a drug that is only slightly different than an FDA-approved drug that is commercially available. In these circumstances, FDA will consider whether there is documentation of the medical need for the particular variation of the compound for the particular patient; and
- Failing to operate in conformance with applicable state law regulating the practice of pharmacy.

Compounding

USP defines stability of an oral liquid formulation as "the extent to which the preparation retains, within specified limits, and throughout its period of storage and use, the same properties and characteristics that it possessed at the time of compounding.[2] When evaluating the stability of a formulation, its chemical, physical, and microbiological stability must be considered. In addition to the properties of the ingredients used to compound the formulation, temperature, radiation, light, air, and humidity are environmental factors that can affect the stability of an extemporaneous formulation. The overall stability of an extemporaneously prepared formulation can also be affected by particle size, pH, the water and solvents used, the container used, and the presence of other chemicals.[3] For this reason, alterations of the formulations listed in this handbook are strongly discouraged. The addition of flavoring agents may affect the pH and other chemical properties of the formulation, hence affecting the shelf life of the formulation. Therefore, if a flavoring agent is needed, it should be added to the dose of the medication immediately before its administration. Flavoring agents should not be added to the entire bottle of the elixir, solution, or suspension unless testing has been performed to confirm the overall stability of the formulation.

The following is a brief description of the preparation methods and techniques, as well as packaging and storage requirements of extemporaneously prepared formulations.

Definitions

Levigating agent—A levigating agent is used to moisten and soften a tablet to facilitate the preparation of a liquid, especially when a large number of tablets is required or the tablets are extremely difficult to crush. Preferably, the vehicle or base solution used for the product is used as the levigating agent.

Suspending agent—A suspending agent is used to prevent agglomeration of the dispersed particles and to increase the viscosity of the liquid. This allows for slow settling of the drug particles to ensure uniform distribution and accurate measurement of the dose.

Elixir—An elixir is a clear, sweetened, alcohol-containing solution that is used mainly for drugs that are insoluble in water alone. It is usually not as sweet and less viscous than a syrup. The alcohol content of elixirs makes it a less desirable vehicle or base solution for preparing extemporaneous formulations in pediatric patients.

Solution—A solution is a liquid containing medication that is dissolved in water or other liquids.

Suspension—A suspension is a dispersion containing fine insoluble particles suspended in a liquid medium.

Syrup—A syrup is a concentrated solution of sugar, such as sucrose in water or other aqueous liquid used as a vehicle or base solution to mask the taste of drugs. The high concentration of sugar in syrups provides preservative property as well.

Simple syrup—Simple syrup is a sucrose solution that is made with purified water alone.

Preparation Methods

The preparation methods of extemporaneous formulations are often determined by the source of the ingredients in the formulation (i.e., injectable, tablet or capsule, and oral liquid). In general, an injectable drug can be measured accurately by a syringe. Oral liquid should be measured using a graduated cylinder. Graduations on dispensing bottles are not accurate and should not be used as a measuring device unless they are calibrated.

When using tablets or capsules to prepare a formulation, the tablets or capsules must be thoroughly and uniformly pulverized by trituration. Trituration is a process in which substances are reduced to fine particles in a mortar with a pestle. Small particles are more easily dispersed throughout the vehicle or base solution, settle less quickly, and are less likely to cake once they settle. Therefore, particles to be suspended in the vehicle or base solution must be small and uniform to ensure consistency and accuracy of dosing. Once triturated, the powder should be levigated with a levigating agent. The levigating agent is selected on the basis of its ability to form a smooth paste with the powder to be levigated and on its compatibility with the substance. The vehicle or base solution should be added to the paste in increasing amounts and mixed thoroughly.

The mixture should be transferred to a graduated cylinder. A small amount of vehicle or base solution should be used to rinse the mortar and the solution then poured into the graduated cylinder. The volume should be adjusted in the graduated cylinder to the quantity required for the formulation. The final product should be placed in the dispensing container.

Ideally, a light-resistant container should be used to protect the contents. It is also important to ensure that the storage condition of the extemporaneous formulations is appropriate. Refrigerator temperature should be maintained between 2°C to 8°C (36°F to 45°F) for formulations that require refrigeration. Formulations to be stored at room temperature should be maintained between 20°C to 25°C (68°F to 77°F).

For a comprehensive overview of necessary considerations when preparing extemporaneous formulations, please refer to the ASHP Technical Assistance Bulletin on Compounding Nonsterile Products in Pharmacies (Appendix A) and the ASHP Guidelines on Pharmacy-Prepared Ophthalmic Products (Appendix B).

References

1. Compliance Policy Guidance for FDA Staff and Industry Sec. 460.200 Pharmacy Compounding. Available at: http://www.fda.gov/ICECI/ComplianceManuals/CompliancePolicyGuidanceManual/ucm074398.htm. Accessed April 2, 2010.

2. *USP Pharmacists' Pharmacopeia.* 2nd ed. Rockville, MD: The United States Pharmacopeia Convention Inc; 2008–2009.

3. Allen LV Jr. *The Art, Science, and Technology of Pharmaceutical Compounding.* 3rd ed. Washington, DC: American Pharmacists Association; 2008.

Elixir/Solution/Suspension/Syrup

Acetazolamide Suspension 25 mg/ml

Ingredients:

Acetazolamide 250-mg tablet   12 tablets

Ora-Sweet/Ora-Plus*   **QSAD:** 120 ml

Preparation Details:

1. Triturate tablets to a fine powder in a mortar and pestle.
2. Levigate with a small amount of base solution to form a paste.
3. Add base solution in increasing amounts while mixing thoroughly.
4. Transfer contents of the mortar to a graduated cylinder.
5. Rinse the mortar and pestle with base solution and pour into graduated cylinder.
6. Add base solution to the graduated cylinder to achieve the total volume indicated above.
7. Transfer contents of the graduated cylinder into an appropriate size amber bottle.
8. Shake well to mix.

Storage Conditions: Room Temperature or Refrigerate

Special Instructions: *Mix 60 ml of Ora-Sweet with 60 ml of Ora-Plus. Use mixture as base solution. Shake well before use.

Alternatives: May substitute base solution with cherry syrup or 60 ml of Ora-Sweet SF mixed with 60 ml of Ora-Plus.

Study Container Type: Plastic

Expiration Date: 60 days

References

1. Allen Jr LV, Erickson III MA. Stability of acetazolamide, allopurinol, azathioprine, clonazepam, and flucytosine in extemporaneously compounded oral liquids. *Am J Health-Syst Pharm.* 1996;53:1944–1999.

Allopurinol Suspension 20 mg/ml

Ingredients:

Allopurinol 300-mg tablet	8 tablets
Ora-Sweet/Ora-Plus*	**QSAD:** 120 ml

Preparation Details:

1. Triturate tablets to a fine powder in a mortar and pestle.
2. Levigate with a small amount of base solution to form a paste.
3. Add base solution in increasing amounts while mixing thoroughly.
4. Transfer contents of the mortar to a graduated cylinder.
5. Rinse the mortar and pestle with base solution and pour into graduated cylinder.
6. Add base solution to the graduated cylinder to achieve the total volume indicated above.
7. Transfer contents of the graduated cylinder into an appropriate size amber bottle.
8. Shake well to mix.

Storage Conditions: Room Temperature or Refrigerate

Special Instructions: *Mix 60 ml of Ora-Sweet with 60 ml of Ora-Plus. Use mixture as base solution. Shake well before use.

Alternatives: May substitute base solution with cherry syrup or 60 ml of Ora-Sweet SF mixed with 60 ml of Ora-Plus.

Study Container Type: Plastic

Expiration Date: 60 days

References

1. Allen Jr LV, Erickson III MA. Stability of acetazolamide, allopurinol, azathioprine, clonazepam, and flucytosine in extemporaneously compounded oral liquids. *Am J Health-Syst Pharm.* 1996;53:1944–1999.

Amiodarone Suspension 5 mg/ml

Ingredients:

Amiodarone 200-mg tablet	3 tablets
Sodium Bicarbonate 8.4%	4 ml
Ora-Sweet/Ora-Plus*	**QSAD:** 120 ml

Preparation Details:

1. Triturate tablets to a fine powder in a mortar and pestle.
2. Levigate with a small amount of base solution to form a paste.
3. Add base solution in increasing amounts while mixing thoroughly.
4. Transfer contents of the mortar to a graduated cylinder.
5. Rinse the mortar and pestle with base solution and pour into graduated cylinder.
6. Add base solution to the graduated cylinder to achieve the total volume indicated above.
7. Transfer contents of the graduated cylinder into an appropriate size amber bottle.
8. Shake well to mix.

Storage Conditions: Refrigerate

Special Instructions: *Mix 60 ml of Ora-Sweet with 60 ml of Ora-Plus. Add approximately 4 ml of Sodium Bicarbonate 8.4% to adjust pH of mixture to 6–7. Use mixture as base solution. Expiration date of 42 days when stored in room temperature. Shake well before use.

Alternatives: May substitute base solution with 60 ml of Ora-Sweet SF mixed with 60 ml of Ora-Plus and adjust pH to 6–7 with Sodium Bicarbonate 8.4% as above or with 60 ml of Methylcellulose 1% (see page 60 for preparation directions) mixed with 60 ml of Simple Syrup NF.

Study Container Type: Plastic

Expiration Date: 90 days

References

1. Nahata MC, Morosco RS, Hipple TF. Stability of amiodarone in extemporaneous oral suspensions prepared from commercially available vehicles. *J Pediatr Pharm Pract.* 1999;4:186–189.

2. Nahata MC. Stability of amiodarone in an oral suspension stored under refrigeration and at room temperature. *Ann Pharmacother.* 1997;31:851–852.

Amitriptyline Syrup 1 mg/ml

Ingredients:

Amitriptyline 25-mg tablet	4 tablets
Glycerin USP	2 ml
Simple Syrup	**QSAD:** 100 ml

Preparation Details:

1. Triturate tablets to a fine powder in a mortar and pestle.
2. Levigate with glycerin to form a paste.
3. Add base solution in increasing amounts while mixing thoroughly.
4. Transfer contents of the mortar to a graduated cylinder.
5. Rinse the mortar and pestle with base solution and pour into graduated cylinder.
6. Add base solution to the graduated cylinder to achieve the total volume indicated above.
7. Transfer contents of the graduated cylinder into an appropriate size amber bottle.
8. Shake well to mix.

Storage Conditions: Room Temperature

Special Instructions: Shake well before use.

Study Container Type: Glass

Expiration Date: 21 days

References

1. Gupta VD. Chemical stability of amitriptyline hydrochloride in oral liquid dosage forms. *Int J Pharm Compound.* 2009;13:445–456.

Amlodipine Suspension 1 mg/ml

Ingredients:

Amlodipine 5-mg tablet	24 tablets
Ora-Sweet/Ora-Plus*	**QSAD:** 120 ml

Preparation Details:

1. Triturate tablets to a fine powder in a mortar and pestle.
2. Levigate with a small amount of base solution to form a paste.
3. Add base solution in increasing amounts while mixing thoroughly.
4. Transfer contents of the mortar to a graduated cylinder.
5. Rinse the mortar and pestle with base solution and pour into graduated cylinder.
6. Add base solution to the graduated cylinder to achieve the total volume indicated above.
7. Transfer contents of the graduated cylinder into an appropriate size amber bottle.
8. Shake well to mix.

Storage Conditions: Refrigerate

Special Instructions: *Mix 60 ml of Ora-Sweet with 60 ml of Ora-Plus. Use mixture as base solution. Expiration date of 56 days when stored at room temperature. Shake well before use.

Alternatives: May substitute base solution with 60 ml of Methylcellulose 1% (see page 60 for preparation directions) mixed with 60 ml of Simple Syrup NF.

Study Container Type: Plastic

Expiration Date: 90 days

References

1. Nahata MC, Morosco RS, Hipple TF. Stability of amlodipine besylate in two liquid dosage forms. *J Am Pharm Assoc.* 1999;39:375–377.

Amphetamine and Dextroamphetamine (Adderall) Suspension 1 mg/ml

Ingredients:

Amphetamine and dextroamphetamine (Adderall) 10-mg tablet	12 tablets
Ora-Sweet/Ora-Plus*	**QSAD:** 120 ml

Preparation Details:

1. Triturate tablets to a fine powder in a mortar and pestle.
2. Levigate with a small amount of base solution to form a paste.
3. Add base solution in increasing amounts while mixing thoroughly.
4. Transfer contents of the mortar to a graduated cylinder.
5. Rinse the mortar and pestle with base solution and pour into graduated cylinder.
6. Add base solution to the graduated cylinder to achieve the total volume indicated above.
8. Shake well to mix.

Storage Conditions: Room Temperature

Special Instructions: *Mix 60 ml of Ora-Sweet with 60 ml of Ora-Plus. Use mixture as base solution. Shake well before use.

Alternatives: May substitute base solution with Ora-Sweet alone or Ora-Plus alone.

Study Container Type: Glass

Expiration Date: 30 days

References

1. Justice J, Kupiec TC, Matthews P, et al. Stability of Adderall in extemporaneously compounded oral liquids. *Am J Health-Syst Pharm.* 2001;58:1418–1421.

Atenolol Syrup 2 mg/ml–Formulation 1

Ingredients:

Atenolol 25-mg tablet   12 tablets

Oral Diluent (Roxane)   **QSAD:** 150 ml

Preparation Details:

1. Triturate tablets to a fine powder in a mortar and pestle.
2. Levigate with a small amount of base solution to form a paste.
3. Add base solution in increasing amounts while mixing thoroughly.
4. Transfer contents of the mortar to a graduated cylinder.
5. Rinse the mortar and pestle with base solution and pour into graduated cylinder.
6. Add base solution to the graduated cylinder to achieve the total volume indicated above.
7. Transfer contents of the graduated cylinder into an appropriate size amber bottle.
8. Shake well to mix.

Storage Conditions: Room Temperature or Refrigerate

Special Instructions: Shake well before use.

Study Container Type: Glass

Expiration Date: 40 days

References

1. Garner SS, Wiest DB, Reynolds Jr ER. Stability of atenolol in an extemporaneously compounded oral liquid. *Am J Hosp Pharm.* 1994;51:508–511.

Atenolol Syrup 2 mg/ml–Formulation 2

Ingredients:

Atenolol 25-mg tablet	12 tablets
Glycerin USP	2 ml
Ora-Sweet SF	**QSAD:** 150 ml

Preparation Details:

1. Triturate tablets to a fine powder in a mortar and pestle.
2. Levigate with a small amount of glycerin to form a paste.
3. Add base solution in increasing amounts while mixing thoroughly.
4. Transfer contents of the mortar to a graduated cylinder.
5. Rinse the mortar and pestle with base solution and pour into graduated cylinder.
6. Add base solution to the bottle to achieve the total volume indicated above.
7. Transfer contents of the graduated cylinder into an appropriate size amber bottle.
8. Shake well to mix.

Storage Conditions: Room Temperature

Special Instructions: Shake well before use.

Study Container Type: Unknown

Expiration Date: 90 days

References

1. Patel D, Doshi DH, Desai A. Short-term stability of atenolol in oral liquid formulations. *Int J Pharm Compound.* 1997;1:437–439.

Azathioprine Suspension 50 mg/ml

Ingredients:

Azathioprine 50-mg tablet   120 tablets

Ora-Sweet/Ora-Plus*   **QSAD:** 120 ml

Preparation Details:

1. Triturate tablets to a fine powder in a mortar and pestle.
2. Levigate with a small amount of base solution to form a paste.
3. Add base solution in increasing amounts while mixing thoroughly.
4. Transfer contents of the mortar to a graduated cylinder.
5. Rinse the mortar and pestle with base solution and pour into graduated cylinder.
6. Add base solution to the graduated cylinder to achieve the total volume indicated above.
7. Transfer contents of the graduated cylinder into an appropriate size amber bottle.
8. Shake well to mix.

Storage Conditions: Room Temperature or Refrigerate

Special Instructions: *Mix 60 ml of Ora-Sweet with 60 ml of Ora-Plus. Use mixture as base solution. Shake well before use.

Alternatives: May substitute base solution with cherry syrup or 60 ml of Ora-Sweet SF mixed with 60 ml of Ora-Plus.

Study Container Type: Plastic

Expiration Date: 60 days

References

1. Allen Jr LV, Erickson III MA. Stability of acetazolamide, allopurinol, azathioprine, clonazepam, and flucytosine in extemporaneously compounded oral liquids. *Am J Health-Syst Pharm.* 1996;53:1944–1999.

Baclofen Suspension 10 mg/ml

Ingredients:

Baclofen 20-mg tablet   60 tablets

Ora-Sweet/Ora-Plus*   **QSAD:** 120 ml

Preparation Details:

1. Triturate tablets to a fine powder in a mortar and pestle.
2. Levigate with a small amount of base solution to form a paste.
3. Add base solution in increasing amounts while mixing thoroughly.
4. Transfer contents of the mortar to a graduated cylinder.
5. Rinse the mortar and pestle with base solution and pour into graduated cylinder.
6. Add base solution to the graduated cylinder to achieve the total volume indicated above.
7. Transfer contents of the graduated cylinder into an appropriate size amber bottle.
8. Shake well to mix.

Storage Conditions: Room Temperature or Refrigerate

Special Instructions: *Mix 60 ml of Ora-Sweet with 60 ml of Ora-Plus. Use mixture as base solution. Shake well before use.

Alternatives: May substitute base solution with cherry syrup or 60 ml of Ora-Sweet SF mixed with 60 ml of Ora-Plus.

Study Container Type: Plastic

Expiration Date: 60 days

References

1. Allen Jr LV, Erickson III MA. Stability of baclofen, captopril, diltiazem hydrochloride, dipyridamole, and flecainide acetate in extemporaneously compounded oral liquids. *Am J Health-Syst Pharm.* 1996;53:2179–2184.

Baclofen Syrup 5 mg/ml

Ingredients:

Baclofen 20-mg tablet	30 tablets
Glycerin USP	Small amount
Simple Syrup	**QSAD:** 120 ml

Preparation Details:

1. Triturate tablets to a fine powder in a mortar and pestle.
2. Levigate with a small amount of Glycerin to form a paste.
3. Add base solution in increasing amounts while mixing thoroughly.
4. Transfer contents of the mortar to a graduated cylinder.
5. Rinse the mortar and pestle with base solution and pour into graduated cylinder.
6. Add base solution to the graduated cylinder to achieve the total volume indicated above.
7. Transfer contents of the graduated cylinder into an appropriate size amber bottle.
8. Shake well to mix.

Storage Conditions: Refrigerate

Special Instructions: Shake well before use.

Study Container Type: Glass

Expiration Date: 35 days

References

1. Johnson CE, Hart SM. Stability of an extemporaneously compounded baclofen oral liquid. *Am J Hosp Pharm.* 1993;50:2353–2355.

Bethanechol Solution 1 mg/ml

Ingredients:

Bethanechol 10-mg tablet   12 tablets

Sterile Water for Irrigation   **QSAD:** 120 ml

Preparation Details:

1. Triturate tablets to a fine powder in a mortar and pestle.
2. Levigate with a small amount of base solution to form a paste.
3. Add base solution in increasing amounts while mixing thoroughly.
4. Transfer contents of the mortar to a graduated cylinder.
5. Rinse the mortar and pestle with base solution and pour into graduated cylinder.
6. Add base solution to the graduated cylinder to achieve the total volume indicated above.
7. Transfer contents of the graduated cylinder into an appropriate size amber bottle.
8. Shake well to mix.

Storage Conditions: Refrigerate

Special Instructions: Shake well before use.

Study Container Type: Glass

Expiration Date: 30 days

References

1. Schlatter JL, Saulnier JL. Bethanechol chloride oral solutions: stability and use in infants. *Ann Pharmacother.* 1997;31:294–296.

Bethanechol Suspension 5 mg/ml

Ingredients:

Bethanechol 10-mg tablet	60 tablets
Ora-Sweet/Ora-Plus*	**QSAD:** 120 ml

Preparation Details:

1. Triturate tablets to a fine powder in a mortar and pestle.
2. Levigate with a small amount of base solution to form a paste.
3. Add base solution in increasing amounts while mixing thoroughly.
4. Transfer contents of the mortar to a graduated cylinder.
5. Rinse the mortar and pestle with base solution and pour into graduated cylinder.
6. Add base solution to the graduated cylinder to achieve the total volume indicated above.
7. Transfer contents of the graduated cylinder into an appropriate size amber bottle.
8. Shake well to mix.

Storage Conditions: Room Temperature or Refrigerate

Special Instructions: *Mix 60 ml of Ora-Sweet with 60 ml of Ora-Plus. Use mixture as base solution. Shake well before use.

Alternatives: May substitute base solution with cherry syrup or 60 ml of Ora-Sweet SF mixed with 60 ml of Ora-Plus.

Study Container Type: Plastic

Expiration Date: 60 days

References

1. Allen Jr LV, Erickson III MA. Stability of bethanechol chloride, pyrazinamide, quinidine sulfate, rifampin, and tetracycline hydrochloride in extemporaneously compounded oral liquids. *Am J Health-Syst Pharm.* 1998;55:1804–1809.

Busulfan Syrup 2 mg/ml

Ingredients:

Busulfan 2-mg tablet	120 tablets
Simple Syrup	**QSAD:** 120 ml

Preparation Details:

Must be prepared in a vertical hood. Must wear mask during preparation.

1. Triturate tablets to a fine powder in a mortar and pestle.
2. Levigate with a small amount of base solution to form a paste.
3. Add base solution in increasing amounts while mixing thoroughly.
4. Transfer contents of the mortar to a graduated cylinder.
5. Rinse the mortar and pestle with base solution and pour into graduated cylinder.
6. Add base solution to the graduated cylinder to achieve the total volume indicated above.
7. Transfer contents of the graduated cylinder into an appropriate size amber bottle.
8. Shake well to mix.

Storage Conditions: Refrigerate

Special Instructions: Shake well before use. Caution chemo-therapy.

Study Container Type: Unknown

Expiration Date: 30 days

References

1. Partin JM, Poust RI, Cox FP. Stability of busulfan in suspension. *Pharmaceutical Research.* 1988;5:S–74.

2. Allen Jr LV. Busulfan oral suspension. *US Pharmacist.* 1990;15:94–95

Captopril Solution 1 mg/ml—Formulation 1

Ingredients:

Captopril 12.5-mg tablet	8 tablets
Sodium Ascorbate injection	500 mg
Sterile Water for Irrigation	**QSAD:** 100 ml

Preparation Details:

1. Place tablets in graduated cylinder.
2. Add Sterile Water for Irrigation slowly while dissolution occurs.
3. Add Sodium Ascorbate injection to graduated cylinder.
4. Add remaining Sterile Water for Irrigation to the graduated cylinder to achieve the total volume indicated above.
5. Transfer the solution into an appropriate size amber bottle.
6. Shake well to mix.

Storage Conditions: Refrigerate

Special Instructions: Expiration date of 14 days when stored at room temperature. Shake well before use.

Alternatives: May substitute additive with ascorbic acid 500-mg tablet. Formulation without Sodium Ascorbate injection or ascorbic acid tablet has expiration date of 14 days refrigerated and 7 days when stored at room temperature.

Study Container Type: Glass

Expiration Date: 56 days

References

1. Nahata MC, Morosco RS, Hipple TF. Stability of captopril in three liquid dosage forms. *Am J Hosp Pharm*. 1994;51:95–96.

2. Nahata MC, Morosco R, Hipple TF. Stability of captopril in liquid containing ascorbic acid or sodium ascorbate. *Am J Hosp Pharm*. 1994;51:1707–1708.

Captopril Suspension 0.75 mg/ml

Ingredients:

Captopril 12.5-mg tablet	6 tablets
Ora-Sweet/Ora-Plus*	**QSAD:** 100 ml

Preparation Details:

1. Triturate tablets to a fine powder in a mortar and pestle.
2. Levigate with a small amount of base solution to form a paste.
3. Add base solution in increasing amounts while mixing thoroughly.
4. Transfer contents of the mortar to a graduated cylinder.
5. Rinse the mortar and pestle with base solution and pour into graduated cylinder.
6. Add base solution to the graduated cylinder to achieve the total volume indicated above.
7. Transfer contents of the graduated cylinder into an appropriate size amber bottle.
8. Shake well to mix.

Storage Conditions: Refrigerate

Special Instructions: *Mix 60 ml of Ora-Sweet with 60 ml of Ora-Plus. Use mixture as base solution. Expiration date of 7 days when stored at room temperature. Shake well before use.

Alternatives: May substitute base solution with 60 ml of Ora-Sweet SF mixed with 60 ml of Ora-Plus with expiration date of 10 days when refrigerated and 5 days when stored at room temperature.

Study Container Type: Plastic

Expiration Date: 14 days

References

1. Allen Jr LV, Erickson III MA. Stability of baclofen, captopril, diltiazem hydrochloride, dipyridamole, and flecainide acetate in extemporaneously compounded oral liquids. *Am J Health-Syst Pharm.* 1996;53:2179–2184.

Captopril Suspension 1 mg/ml—Formulation 2

Ingredients:

Captopril 12.5-mg tablet   8 tablets

Simple Syrup NF/Methylcellulose 1%*   **QSAD:** 100 ml

Preparation Details:

1. Triturate tablets to a fine powder in a mortar and pestle.
2. Levigate with a small amount of base solution to form a paste.
3. Add base solution in increasing amounts while mixing thoroughly.
4. Transfer contents of the mortar to a graduated cylinder.
5. Rinse the mortar and pestle with base solution and pour into graduated cylinder.
6. Add base solution to the graduated cylinder to achieve the total volume indicated above.
7. Transfer contents of the graduated cylinder into an appropriate size amber bottle.
8. Shake well to mix.

Storage Conditions: Room Temperature or Refrigerate

Special Instructions: *Mix 50 ml of Simple Syrup NF with 50 ml of Methylcellulose 1%. Use mixture as base solution. Shake well before use.

Study Container Type: Glass

Expiration Date: 7 days

References

1. Nahata MC, Morosco RS, Hipple TF. Stability of captopril in three liquid dosage forms. *Am J Hosp Pharm.* 1994;51:95–96.

Carvedilol Suspension 0.1 mg/ml

Ingredients:

Carvedilol 3.125-mg tablet	4 tablets
Sterile Water for Irrigation	20 ml
Ora-Plus	60 ml
Ora-Sweet	**QSAD:** 125 ml

Preparation Details:

1. Triturate tablets to a fine powder in a mortar and pestle.
2. Levigate with Sterile Water for Irrigation to form a paste.
3. Add Ora-Plus in increasing amounts while mixing thoroughly.
4. Transfer contents of the mortar to a graduated cylinder.
5. Rinse the mortar and pestle with base solution and pour into graduated cylinder.
6. Add base solution to the graduated cylinder to achieve the total volume indicated above.
7. Transfer contents of the graduated cylinder into an appropriate size amber bottle.
8. Shake well to mix.

Storage Conditions: Room Temperature

Special Instructions: Shake well before use.

Study Container Type: Glass

Expiration Date: 84 days

References

1. Data on file 2007. Philadelphia PA: GlaxoSmithKline; EC2007/00022/01.
2. Data on file 2007. Philadelphia PA: GlaxoSmithKline; EC2007/00010/00.

Carvedilol Suspension 1.67 mg/ml

Ingredients:

Carvedilol 25-mg tablet	8 tablets
Sterile Water for Irrigation	20 ml
Ora-Plus	60 ml
Ora-Sweet	**QSAD:** 120 ml

Preparation Details:

1. Triturate tablets to a fine powder in a mortar and pestle.
2. Levigate with Sterile Water for Irrigation to form a paste.
3. Add Ora-Plus in increasing amounts while mixing thoroughly.
4. Transfer contents of the mortar to a graduated cylinder.
5. Rinse the mortar and pestle with base solution and pour into graduated cylinder.
6. Add base solution to the graduated cylinder to achieve the total volume indicated above.
7. Transfer contents of the graduated cylinder into an appropriate size amber bottle.
8. Shake well to mix.

Storage Conditions: Room Temperature

Special Instructions: Shake well before use.

Study Container Type: Glass

Expiration Date: 84 days

References

1. Data on file 2007. Philadelphia PA: GlaxoSmithKline; EC2007/00022/01.
2. Data on file 2007. Philadelphia PA: GlaxoSmithKline; EC2007/00010/00.

Chloroquine Phosphate Suspension 15 mg/ml

Ingredients:

Chloroquine Phosphate 500-mg tablet	3 tablets
Ora-Sweet/Ora-Plus*	**QSAD:** 100 ml

Preparation Details:

1. Remove film coating off tablets with a wet paper towel.
2. Triturate tablets to a fine powder in a mortar and pestle.
3. Levigate with a small amount of base solution to form a paste.
4. Add base solution in increasing amounts while mixing thoroughly.
5. Transfer contents of the mortar to a graduated cylinder.
6. Rinse the mortar and pestle with base solution and pour into graduated cylinder.
7. Add base solution to the graduated cylinder to achieve the total volume indicated above.
8. Transfer contents of the graduated cylinder into an appropriate size amber bottle.
9. Shake well to mix.

Storage Conditions: Room Temperature or Refrigerate

Special Instructions: *Mix 50 ml of Ora-Sweet with 50 ml of Ora-Plus. Use mixture as base solution. Chloroquine Phosphate 15 mg/ml = Chloroquine Base 9 mg/ml. Chloroquine Phosphate 500 mg = Chloroquine Base 300 mg. Shake well before use.

Alternatives: May substitute base solution with cherry syrup or 50 ml of Ora-Sweet SF mixed with 50 ml of Ora-Plus.

Study Container Type: Plastic

Expiration Date: 60 days

References

1. Allen Jr LV, Erickson III MA. Stability of alprazolam, chloroquine phosphate, cisapride, enalapril maleate, and hydralazine hydrochloride in extemporaneously compounded oral liquids. *Am J Health-Syst Pharm.* 1998;55:1915–1920.

Chloroquine Phosphate Syrup 16.7 mg/ml

Ingredients:

Chloroquine Phosphate 500-mg tablet	4 tablets
Sterile Water for Irrigation	Small amount
Cherry Syrup	**QSAD:** 120 ml

Preparation Details:

1. Remove film coating off tablets with a wet paper towel.
2. Triturate tablets to a fine powder in a mortar and pestle.
3. Levigate with Sterile Water for Irrigation to form a paste.
4. Add base solution in increasing amounts while mixing thoroughly.
5. Transfer contents of the mortar to a graduated cylinder.
6. Rinse the mortar and pestle with base solution and pour into graduated cylinder.
7. Add base solution to the graduated cylinder to achieve the total volume indicated above.
8. Transfer contents of the graduated cylinder into an appropriate size amber bottle.
9. Shake well to mix.

Storage Conditions: Room Temperature or Refrigerate

Special Instructions: Chloroquine Phosphate 16.7 mg/ml = Chloroquine Base 10 mg/ml. Chloroquine Phosphate 500 mg = Chloroquine Base 300 mg. Shake well before use.

Study Container Type: Glass

Expiration Date: 28 days

References

1. Mirochnick M, Barnett E, Clarke DF. Stability of chloroquine in an extemporaneously prepared suspension stored at three temperatures. *Pediatr Infect Dis J.* 1994;13:827–828.

Clonazepam Suspension 0.1 mg/ml

Ingredients:

Clonazepam 1-mg tablet	12 tablets
Ora-Sweet/Ora-Plus*	**QSAD:** 120 ml

Preparation Details:

1. Triturate tablets to a fine powder in a mortar and pestle.
2. Levigate with a small amount of base solution to form a paste.
3. Add base solution in increasing amounts while mixing thoroughly.
4. Transfer contents of the mortar to a graduated cylinder.
5. Rinse the mortar and pestle with base solution and pour into graduated cylinder.
6. Add base solution to the graduated cylinder to achieve the total volume indicated above.
7. Transfer contents of the graduated cylinder into an appropriate size amber bottle.
8. Shake well to mix.

Storage Conditions: Room Temperature or Refrigerate

Special Instructions: *Mix 60 ml of Ora-Sweet with 60 ml of Ora-Plus. Use mixture as base solution. Shake well before use.

Alternatives: May substitute base solution with cherry syrup or 60 ml of Ora-Sweet SF mixed with 60 ml of Ora-Plus.

Study Container Type: Plastic

Expiration Date: 60 days

References

1. Allen Jr LV, Erickson III MA. Stability of acetazolamide, allopurinol, azathioprine, clonazepam, and flucytosine in extemporaneously compounded oral liquids. *Am J Health-Syst Pharm.* 1996;53:1944–1949.

Clonidine Syrup 0.1 mg/ml

Ingredients:

Clonidine 0.2-mg tablet	60 tablets
Sterile Water for Irrigation	4 ml
Simple Syrup NF	**QSAD:** 120 ml

Preparation Details:

1. Triturate tablets to a fine powder in a mortar and pestle.
2. Levigate with Sterile Water for Irrigation to form a paste.
3. Add base solution in increasing amounts while mixing thoroughly.
4. Transfer contents of the mortar to a graduated cylinder.
5. Rinse the mortar and pestle with base solution and pour into graduated cylinder.
6. Add base solution to the graduated cylinder to achieve the total volume indicated above.
7. Transfer contents of the graduated cylinder into an appropriate size amber bottle.
8. Shake well to mix.

Storage Conditions: Refrigerate

Special Instructions: Shake well before use.

Study Container Type: Glass

Expiration Date: 28 days

References

1. Levinson ML, Johnson CE. Stability of an extemporaneously compounded clonidine hydrochloride oral liquid. *Am J Hosp Pharm.* 1992;49:122–125.

Clopidogrel Suspension 5 mg/ml

Ingredients:

Clopidogrel 75-mg tablet   8 tablets

Ora-Sweet/Ora-Plus*   **QSAD:** 120 ml

Preparation Details:

1. Triturate tablets to a fine powder in a glass mortar and pestle.
2. Levigate with a small amount of base solution to form a paste.
3. Add base solution in increasing amounts while mixing thoroughly.
4. Transfer contents of the mortar to a graduated cylinder.
5. Rinse the mortar and pestle with base solution and pour into graduated cylinder.
6. Add base solution to the graduated cylinder to achieve the total volume indicated above.
7. Transfer contents of the graduated cylinder into an appropriate size amber bottle.
8. Shake well to mix.

Storage Conditions: Room Temperature or Refrigerate

Special Instructions: *Mix 60 ml of Ora-Sweet with 60 ml of Ora-Plus. Use mixture as base solution. Shake well before use.

Study Container Type: Plastic

Expiration Date: 60 days

References

1. Skillman KL, Caruthers RL, Johnson CE. Stability of an extemporaneously prepared clopidogrel oral suspension. *Am J Health-Syst Pharm*. 2010;67:559–561.

Cyclophosphamide Elixir 2 mg/ml

Ingredients:

Cyclophosphamide 100-mg injection vial	1 vial
Sterile Water for Injection	5 ml
Aromatic Elixir*	**QSAD:** 50 ml

Preparation Details:

Must be prepared in a vertical hood. Must wear mask during preparation.

1. Reconstitute injectable powder with 5 ml of Sterile Water for Injection.
2. Withdraw volume of injectable solution using a 5-ml syringe.
3. Transfer the solution to a graduated cylinder.
4. Add base solution to the graduated cylinder to achieve the total volume indicated above.
5. Transfer contents of the graduated cylinder into an appropriate size amber bottle.
6. Shake well to mix.

Storage Conditions: Refrigerate

Special Instructions: *To prepare Aromatic Elixir, refer to *Remington's Pharmaceutical Sciences,* 18th ed. Easton, PA: Mack Publishing Company; 1990. Shake well before use. Caution chemotherapy.

Study Container Type: Glass

Expiration Date: 14 days

References

1. Brooke D, Davis RE, Bequette RJ. Chemical stability of cyclophosphamide in aromatic elixir USP. *Am J Hosp Pharm.* 1973;30:618–620.

Dantrolene Syrup 5 mg/ml

Ingredients:

Dantrolene 25-mg capsule	20 capsules
Citric Acid Monohydrate	150 mg
Methyl Hydroxybenzoate	150 mg
Sterile Water for Irrigation	10 ml
Simple Syrup NF	**QSAD:** 100 ml

Preparation Details:

1. Open capsules and empty contents into a mortar.
2. Add Citric Acid and Methyl Hydroxybenzoate powder to the mortar.
3. Triturate contents to a fine powder.
4. Levigate with Sterile Water for Irrigation to form a paste.
5. Add base solution in increasing amounts while mixing thoroughly.
6. Transfer contents of the mortar to a graduated cylinder.
7. Rinse the mortar and pestle with base solution and pour into graduated cylinder.
8. Add base solution to the graduated cylinder to achieve the total volume indicated above.
9. Transfer contents of the graduated cylinder into an appropriate size amber bottle.
10. Shake well to mix.

Storage Conditions: Room Temperature or Refrigerate

Special Instructions: Shake well before use.

Study Container Type: Plastic

Expiration Date: 150 days

References

1. Fawcett JP, Stark G, Tucker IG, et al. Stability of dantrolene oral suspension prepared from capsules. *J Clin Pharm Ther.* 1994;19:349–353.

Dapsone Suspension 2 mg/ml—Formulation 1

Ingredients:

Dapsone 25-mg tablet   8 tablets

Ora-Sweet/Ora-Plus*   **QSAD:** 100 ml

Preparation Details:

1. Triturate tablets to a fine powder in a mortar and pestle.
2. Levigate with a small amount of base solution to form a paste.
3. Add base solution in increasing amounts while mixing thoroughly.
4. Transfer contents of the mortar to a graduated cylinder.
5. Rinse the mortar and pestle with base solution and pour into graduated cylinder.
6. Add base solution to the graduated cylinder to achieve the total volume indicated above.
7. Transfer contents of the graduated cylinder into an appropriate size amber bottle.
8. Shake well to mix.

Storage Conditions: Room Temperature or Refrigerate

Special Instructions: *Mix 50 ml of Ora-Sweet with 50 ml of Ora-Plus. Use mixture as base solution. Shake well before use.

Study Container Type: Plastic

Expiration Date: 90 days

References

1. Nahata MC, Morosco RS, Trowbridge JM. Stability of dapsone in two oral liquid dosage forms. *Ann Pharmacother.* 2000;34:848–850.

Dapsone Syrup 2 mg/ml—Formulation 2

Ingredients:

Dapsone 25-mg tablet	8 tablets
Citric Acid crystals	500 mg
Sterile Water for Irrigation	25 ml
Simple Syrup NF	**QSAD:** 100 ml

Preparation Details:

1. Triturate tablets to a fine powder in a mortar and pestle.
2. Dissolve Citric Acid crystals in the volume of Sterile Water for Irrigation indicated above.
3. Levigate with Citric Acid solution to form paste.
4. Add base solution in increasing amounts while mixing thoroughly.
5. Transfer contents of the mortar to a graduated cylinder.
6. Rinse the mortar and pestle with base solution and pour into graduated cylinder.
7. Add base solution to the graduated cylinder to achieve the total volume indicated above.
8. Transfer contents of the graduated cylinder into an appropriate size amber bottle.
9. Shake well to mix.

Storage Conditions: Room Temperature or Refrigerate

Special Instructions: Shake well before use.

Study Container Type: Plastic

Expiration Date: 90 days

References

1. Nahata MC, Morosco RS, Trowbridge JM. Stability of dapsone in two oral liquid dosage forms. *Ann Pharmacother.* 2000;34:848–850.

Diltiazem Suspension 12 mg/ml

Ingredients:

Diltiazem Hydrochloride 90-mg tablet	16 tablets
Ora-Sweet/Ora-Plus*	**QSAD:** 120 ml

Preparation Details:

1. Triturate tablets to a fine powder in a mortar and pestle.
2. Levigate with a small amount of base solution to form a paste.
3. Add base solution in increasing amounts while mixing thoroughly.
4. Transfer contents of the mortar to a graduated cylinder.
5. Rinse the mortar and pestle with base solution and pour into graduated cylinder.
6. Add base solution to the graduated cylinder to achieve the total volume indicated above.
7. Transfer contents of the graduated cylinder into an appropriate size amber bottle.
8. Shake well to mix.

Storage Conditions: Room Temperature or Refrigerate

Special Instructions: *Mix 60 ml of Ora-Sweet with 60 ml of Ora-Plus. Use mixture as base solution. Shake well before use.

Alternatives: May substitute base solution with cherry syrup or 60 ml of Ora-Sweet SF mixed with 60 ml of Ora-Plus.

Study Container Type: Plastic

Expiration Date: 60 days

References

1. Allen Jr LV, Erickson III MA. Stability of baclofen, captopril, diltiazem hydrochloride, dipyridamole, and flecainide acetate in extemporaneously compounded oral liquids. *Am J Health-Syst Pharm.* 1996;53:2179–2184.

Dipyridamole Suspension 10 mg/ml

Ingredients:

Dipyridamole 50-mg tablet	24 tablets
Ora-Sweet/Ora-Plus*	**QSAD:** 120 ml

Preparation Details:

1. Triturate tablets to a fine powder in a mortar and pestle.
2. Levigate with a small amount of base solution to form a paste.
3. Add base solution in increasing amounts while mixing thoroughly.
4. Transfer contents of the mortar to a graduated cylinder.
5. Rinse the mortar and pestle with base solution and pour into graduated cylinder.
6. Add base solution to the graduated cylinder to achieve the total volume indicated above.
7. Transfer contents of the graduated cylinder into an appropriate size amber bottle.
8. Shake well to mix.

Storage Conditions: Room Temperature or Refrigerate

Special Instructions: *Mix 60 ml of Ora-Sweet with 60 ml of Ora-Plus. Use mixture as base solution. Shake well before use.

Alternatives: May substitute base solution with cherry syrup or 60 ml of Ora-Sweet SF mixed with 60 ml of Ora-Plus.

Study Container Type: Plastic

Expiration Date: 60 days

References

1. Allen Jr LV, Erickson III MA. Stability of baclofen, captopril, diltiazem hydrochloride, dipyridamole, and flecainide acetate in extemporaneously compounded oral liquids. *Am J Health-Syst Pharm.* 1996;53:2179–2184.

Disopyramide Syrup 1 mg/ml

Ingredients:

Disopyramide 100-mg capsule   1 capsule

Cherry Syrup   **QSAD:** 100 ml

Preparation Details:

1. Open capsule and empty contents into a mortar.
2. Triturate contents to a fine powder.
3. Levigate with a small amount of base solution to form a paste.
4. Add base solution in increasing amounts while mixing thoroughly.
5. Transfer contents of the mortar to a graduated cylinder.
6. Rinse the mortar and pestle with base solution and pour into graduated cylinder.
7. Add base solution to the graduated cylinder to achieve the total volume indicated above.
8. Transfer contents of the graduated cylinder into an appropriate size amber bottle.
9. Shake well to mix.

Storage Conditions: Room Temperature or Refrigerate

Special Instructions: Shake well before use.

Study Container Type: Glass

Expiration Date: 28 days

References

1. Mathur LK, Lai PK, Shively CD. Stability of disopyramide phosphate in cherry syrup. *Am J Hosp Pharm.* 1982;39:309–310.

Disopyramide Syrup 10 mg/ml

Ingredients:

Disopyramide 100-mg capsule   10 capsules

Cherry Syrup   **QSAD:** 100 ml

Preparation Details:

1. Open capsules and empty contents into a mortar.
2. Triturate contents to a fine powder.
3. Levigate with a small amount of base solution to form a paste.
4. Add base solution in increasing amounts while mixing thoroughly.
5. Transfer contents of the mortar to a graduated cylinder.
6. Rinse the mortar and pestle with base solution and pour into graduated cylinder.
7. Add base solution to the graduated cylinder to achieve the total volume indicated above.
8. Transfer contents of the graduated cylinder into an appropriate size amber bottle.
9. Shake well to mix.

Storage Conditions: Room Temperature or Refrigerate

Special Instructions: Shake well before use.

Study Container Type: Glass

Expiration Date: 28 days

References

1. Mathur LK, Lai PK, Shively CD. Stability of disopyramide phosphate in cherry syrup. *Am J Hosp Pharm.* 1982;39:309–310.

Dolasetron Suspension 10 mg/ml

Ingredients:

Dolasetron 50-mg tablet   24 tablets

Ora-Plus/Ora-Sweet SF*   **QSAD:** 120 ml

Preparation Details:

1. Triturate tablets to a fine powder in a mortar and pestle.
2. Levigate with a small amount of base solution to form a paste.
3. Add base solution in increasing amounts while mixing thoroughly.
4. Transfer contents of the mortar to a graduated cylinder.
5. Rinse the mortar and pestle with base solution and pour into graduated cylinder.
6. Add base solution to the graduated cylinder to achieve the total volume indicated above.
7. Transfer contents of the graduated cylinder into an appropriate size amber bottle.
8. Shake well to mix.

Storage Conditions: Room Temperature or Refrigerate

Special Instructions: *Mix 60 ml of Ora-Sweet SF with 60 ml of Ora-Plus. Use mixture as base solution. Shake well before use.

Alternatives: May substitute base solution with 60 ml of strawberry syrup mixed with 60 ml of Ora-Plus. Strawberry syrup is prepared by mixing 160 ml of Simple Syrup NF and 30 ml of strawberry fountain syrup.

Study Container Type: Plastic

Expiration Date: 90 days

References

1. Johnson CE, Wagner DS, Bussard WE. Stability of dolasetron in two oral liquid vehicles. *Am J Health-Syst Pharm.* 2003;60:2242–2244.

Enalapril Suspension 1 mg/ml

Ingredients:

Enalapril 5-mg tablet	24 tablets
Ora-Sweet/Ora-Plus*	**QSAD:** 120 ml

Preparation Details:

1. Triturate tablets to a fine powder in a mortar and pestle.
2. Levigate with a small amount of base solution to form a paste.
3. Add base solution in increasing amounts while mixing thoroughly.
4. Transfer contents of the mortar to a graduated cylinder.
5. Rinse the mortar and pestle with base solution and pour into graduated cylinder.
6. Add base solution to the graduated cylinder to achieve the total volume indicated above.
7. Transfer contents of the graduated cylinder into an appropriate size amber bottle.
8. Shake well to mix.

Storage Conditions: Room Temperature or Refrigerate

Special Instructions: *Mix 60 ml of Ora-Sweet with 60 ml of Ora-Plus. Use mixture as base solution. Shake well before use.

Alternatives: May substitute base solution with cherry syrup or 60 ml of Ora-Sweet SF mixed with 60 ml of Ora-Plus with an expiration date of 60 days stored at room temperature or refrigerated.

Study Container Type: Plastic

Expiration Date: 90 days

References

1. Nahata MC, Morosco RD, Hipple TF. Stability of enalapril maleate in three extemporaneously prepared oral liquids. *Am J Health-Syst Pharm.* 1998;55:1155–1157.

2. Allen Jr LV, Erickson III MA. Stability of alprazolam, chloroquine phosphate, cisapride, enalapril maleate, and hydralazine hydrochloride in extemporaneously compounded oral liquids. *Am J Health-Syst Pharm.* 1998;55:1915–1920.

Ethacrynic Acid Solution 1 mg/ml

Ingredients:

Ethacrynic Acid 25-mg tablet	6 tablets
Alcohol 98%	15 ml
Methylparaben powder	7.5 mg
Propylparaben powder	3 mg
Sodium Hydroxide 0.1 N	qs to pH 7
Sorbitol solution 50%	**QSAD:** 150 ml

Preparation Details:

1. Triturate tablets to a fine powder in a mortar and pestle.
2. Add Methylparaben and Propylparaben powder in the mortar
3. Levigate with Alcohol to form a paste.
4. Add base solution in increasing amounts while mixing thoroughly.
5. Transfer contents of the mortar to a graduated cylinder.
6. Rinse the mortar and pestle with base solution and pour into graduated cylinder.
7. Add adequate amount of Sodium Hydroxide 0.1 N to adjust for a pH of 7.
8. Add base solution to the graduated cylinder to achieve the total volume indicated above.
9. Transfer contents of the graduated cylinder into an appropriate size amber bottle.
10. Shake well to mix.

Storage Conditions: Room Temperature

Special Instructions: Shake well before use.

Study Container Type: Unknown

Expiration Date: 220 days

References

1. Gupta VD, Gibbs CW, Ghanekar AG. Stability of pediatric liquid dosage forms of ethacrynic acid, indomethacin, methyldopate hydrochloride, prednisone and spironolactone. *Am J Hosp Pharm.* 1978;35:1382–1385.

Etoposide Solution 10 mg/ml

Ingredients:

Etoposide 20-mg/ml injection   60 ml

Sodium Chloride 0.9% injection   **QSAD:** 120 ml

Preparation Details:

Must be prepared in a vertical hood. Must wear mask during preparation.

1. Withdraw volume of injectable solution using a 60-ml syringe.
2. Transfer the solution to a graduated cylinder.
3. Add base solution to the graduated cylinder to achieve the total volume indicated above.
4. Transfer contents of the graduated cylinder into an appropriate size amber bottle.
5. Shake well to mix.

Storage Conditions: Room Temperature

Special Instructions: Shake well before use. Caution chemo-therapy.

Study Container Type: Plastic oral syringe

Expiration Date: 22 days

References

1. McLeod HL, Relling MV. Stability of etoposide solution for oral use. *Am J Hosp Pharm.* 1992;49:2784 2785.

Flecainide Acetate Suspension 20 mg/ml

Ingredients:

Flecainide Acetate 100-mg tablet 24 tablets

Ora-Sweet/Ora-Plus* **QSAD:** 120 ml

Preparation Details:

1. Triturate tablets to a fine powder in a mortar and pestle.
2. Levigate with a small amount of base solution to form a paste.
3. Add base solution in increasing amounts while mixing thoroughly.
4. Transfer contents of the mortar to a graduated cylinder.
5. Rinse the mortar and pestle with base solution and pour into graduated cylinder.
6. Add base solution to the graduated cylinder to achieve the total volume indicated above.
7. Transfer contents of the graduated cylinder into an appropriate size amber bottle.
8. Shake well to mix.

Storage Conditions: Room Temperature or Refrigerate

Special Instructions: *Mix 60 ml of Ora-Sweet with 60 ml of Ora-Plus. Use mixture as base solution. Shake well before use.

Alternatives: May substitute base solution with cherry syrup or 60 ml of Ora-Sweet SF mixed with 60 ml of Ora-Plus.

Study Container Type: Plastic

Expiration Date: 60 days

References

1. Allen Jr LV, Erickson III MA. Stability of baclofen, captopril, diltiazem hydrochloride, dipyridamole, and flecainide acetate in extemporaneously compounded oral liquids. *Am J Health-Syst Pharm.* 1996;53:2179–2184.

Flecainide Acetate Syrup 5 mg/ml

Ingredients:

Flecainide Acetate 100-mg tablet   6 tablets

Oral diluent (Roxane)   **QSAD:** 120 ml

Preparation Details:

1. Triturate tablets to a fine powder in a mortar and pestle.
2. Levigate with a small amount of base solution to form a paste.
3. Add base solution in increasing amounts while mixing thoroughly.
4. Transfer contents of the mortar to a graduated cylinder.
5. Rinse the mortar and pestle with base solution and pour into graduated cylinder.
6. Add base solution to the graduated cylinder to achieve the total volume indicated above.
7. Transfer contents of the graduated cylinder into an appropriate size amber bottle.
8. Shake well to mix.

Storage Conditions: Room Temperature or Refrigerate

Special Instructions: Shake well before use.

Study Container Type: Glass

Expiration Date: 45 days

References

1. Wiest DB, Garner SS, Pagacz LR, et al. Stability of flecainide acetate in an extemporaneously compounded oral suspension. *Am J Hosp Pharm.* 1992;49:1467–1470.

Flucytosine Suspension 10 mg/ml

Ingredients:

Flucytosine 250-mg capsule   4 capsules

Ora-Sweet/Ora-Plus*   **QSAD:**100 ml

Preparation Details:

1. Open capsules and empty contents into a mortar.
2. Triturate contents to a fine powder.
3. Levigate with a small amount of base solution to form a paste.
4. Add base solution in increasing amounts while mixing thoroughly.
5. Transfer contents of the mortar to a graduated cylinder.
6. Rinse the mortar and pestle with base solution and pour into graduated cylinder.
7. Add base solution to the graduated cylinder to achieve the total volume indicated above.
8. Transfer contents of the graduated cylinder into an appropriate size amber bottle.
9. Shake well to mix.

Storage Conditions: Room Temperature or Refrigerate

Special Instructions: *Mix 50 ml of Ora-Sweet with 50 ml of Ora-Plus. Use mixture as base solution. Shake well before use.

Alternatives: May substitute base solution with cherry syrup or 50 ml of Ora-Sweet SF mixed with 50 ml of Ora-Plus.

Study Container Type: Plastic

Expiration Date: 60 days

References

1. Allen Jr LV, Erickson III MA. Stability of acetazolamide, allopurinol, azathioprine, clonazepam, and flucytosine in extemporaneously compounded oral liquids. *Am J Health-Syst Pharm.* 1996;53:1944–1999.

Flucytosine Suspension 50 mg/ml

Ingredients:

Flucytosine 250-mg capsule	24 capsules
Ora-Plus/Ora-Sweet SF*	**QSAD:** 120 ml

Preparation Details:

1. Open capsules and empty contents into a mortar.
2. Triturate contents to a fine powder.
3. Levigate with a small amount of base solution to form a paste.
4. Add base solution in increasing amounts while mixing thoroughly.
5. Transfer contents of the mortar to a graduated cylinder.
6. Rinse the mortar and pestle with base solution and pour into graduated cylinder.
7. Add base solution to the graduated cylinder to achieve the total volume indicated above.
8. Transfer contents of the graduated cylinder into an appropriate size amber bottle.
9. Shake well to mix.

Storage Conditions: Room Temperature or Refrigerate

Special Instructions: *Mix 60 ml of Ora-Sweet SF with 60 ml of Ora-Plus. Use mixture as base solution. Shake well before use.

Alternatives: May substitute base solution with 60 ml of strawberry syrup mixed with 60 ml of Ora-Plus. Strawberry syrup is prepared by mixing 160 ml of Simple Syrup NF and 30 ml of strawberry fountain syrup.

Study Container Type: Plastic

Expiration Date: 90 days

References

1. Vandenbussche H, Johnson CE, Yun J, et al. Stability of flucytosine 50 mg/ml in extemporaneous oral liquid formulation. *Am J Health-Syst Pharm*. 2002;59:1853–1855.

Ganciclovir Syrup 100 mg/ml

Ingredients:

Ganciclovir 250-mg capsule   48 capsules

Ora-Sweet   **QSAD:** 120 ml

Preparation Details:

Must be prepared in a vertical hood. Must wear mask during preparation.

1. Open capsules and empty contents into a mortar.
2. Triturate contents to a fine powder.
3. Levigate with a small amount of base solution to form a paste.
4. Add base solution in increasing amounts while mixing thoroughly.
5. Transfer contents of the mortar to a graduated cylinder.
6. Rinse the mortar and pestle with base solution and pour into graduated cylinder.
7. Add base solution to the graduated cylinder to achieve the total volume indicated above.
8. Transfer contents of the graduated cylinder into an appropriate size amber bottle.
9. Shake well to mix.

Storage Conditions: Room Temperature

Special Instructions: Shake well before use. Caution teratogenic agent.

Alternatives: May substitute base solution with Ora-Sweet NF.

Study Container Type: Plastic

Expiration Date: 120 days

References

1. Anaizi NH, Swenson CF, Dentinger PJ. Stability of ganciclovir in extemporaneously compounded oral liquids. *Am J Health-Syst Pharm.* 1999;56:1738–1741.

Hydralazine Suspension 4 mg/ml

Ingredients:

Hydralazine 25-mg tablet	16 tablets
Ora-Plus/Ora-Sweet SF*	**QSAD:**100 ml

Preparation Details:

1. Triturate tablets to a fine powder in a mortar and pestle.
2. Levigate with a small amount of base solution to form a paste.
3. Add base solution in increasing amounts while mixing thoroughly.
4. Transfer contents of the mortar to a graduated cylinder.
5. Rinse the mortar and pestle with base solution and pour into graduated cylinder.
6. Add base solution to the graduated cylinder to achieve the total volume indicated above.
7. Transfer contents of the graduated cylinder into an appropriate size amber bottle.
8. Shake well to mix.

Storage Conditions: Refrigerate

Special Instructions: *Mix 50 ml of Ora-Plus with 50 ml of Ora-Sweet SF. Use mixture as base solution. Shake well before use.

Alternatives: May substitute base solution with 50 ml of Ora-Sweet mixed with 50 ml of Ora-Plus with expiration date of 1 day when refrigerated.

Study Container Type: Plastic

Expiration Date: 2 days

References

1. Allen Jr LV, Erickson III MA. Stability of alprazolam, chloroquine phosphate, cisapride, enalapril maleate, and hydralazine hydrochloride in extemporaneously compounded oral liquids. *Am J Health-Syst Pharm.* 1998;55:1915–1920.

Hydrocortisone Suspension 1 mg/ml

Ingredients:

Hydrocortisone 10-mg tablet   12 tablets

Ora-Sweet/Ora-Plus*   **QSAD:** 120 ml

Preparation Details:

1. Triturate tablets to a fine powder in a mortar and pestle.
2. Levigate with a small amount of base solution to form a paste.
3. Add base solution in increasing amounts while mixing thoroughly.
4. Transfer contents of the mortar to a graduated cylinder.
5. Rinse the mortar and pestle with base solution and pour into graduated cylinder.
6. Add base solution to the graduated cylinder to achieve the total volume indicated above.
7. Transfer contents of the graduated cylinder into an appropriate size amber bottle.
8. Shake well to mix.

Storage Conditions: Room Temperature or Refrigerate

Special Instructions: *Mix 60 ml of Ora-Plus with 60 ml of Ora-Sweet. Use mixture as base solution. Shake well before use.

Study Container Type: Plastic

Expiration Date: 91 days

References

1. Chong G, Decarie D, Ensom MHH. Stability of hydrocortisone in extemporaneously compounded suspension. *J Inform Pharmacother.* 2003;13:100–110.

Hydrocortisone Suspension 2 mg/ml

Ingredients:

Hydrocortisone 10-mg tablet   24 tablets

Ora-Sweet/Ora-Plus*   **QSAD:** 120 ml

Preparation Details:

1. Triturate tablets to a fine powder in a mortar and pestle.
2. Levigate with a small amount of base solution to form a paste.
3. Add base solution in increasing amounts while mixing thoroughly.
4. Transfer contents of the mortar to a graduated cylinder.
5. Rinse the mortar and pestle with base solution and pour into graduated cylinder.
6. Add base solution to the graduated cylinder to achieve the total volume indicated above.
7. Transfer contents of the graduated cylinder into an appropriate size amber bottle.
8. Shake well to mix.

Storage Conditions: Room Temperature or Refrigerate

Special Instructions: *Mix 60 ml of Ora-Plus with 60 ml of Ora-Sweet. Use mixture as base solution. Shake well before use.

Study Container Type: Plastic

Expiration Date: 91 days

References

1. Chong G, Decarie D, Ensom MHH. Stability of hydrocortisone in extemporaneously compounded suspension. *J Inform Pharmacother.* 2003;13:100–110.

Hydroxyurea Syrup 100 mg/ml

Ingredients:

Hydroxyurea 500-mg capsule	24 capsules
Sterile Water for Irrigation	60 ml
Syrpalta, dye-free	**QSAD:** 120 ml

Preparation Details:

Must be prepared in a vertical hood. Must wear mask during preparation.

1. Open capsules and empty contents into a beaker.
2. Add Sterile Water for Irrigation in increasing amounts while mixing thoroughly.
3. Vigorously stir for several hours using a magnetic stirrer.
4. Filter solution to remove insoluble excipients.
5. Transfer contents of the beaker to a graduated cylinder.
6. Rinse the beaker with base solution and pour into graduated cylinder.
7. Add base solution to the graduated cylinder to achieve the total volume indicated above.
8. Transfer contents of the graduated cylinder into an appropriate size amber bottle.
9. Shake well to mix.

Storage Conditions: Room Temperature

Special Instructions: Shake well before use.

Study Container Type: Plastic

Expiration Date: 180 days

References

1. Heeney MM, Whorton MR, Howard TA, et al. Chemical and functional analysis of hydroxyurea oral solutions. *J Pediatr Hematol Oncol.* 2004;26:179–184.

Hypromellose Suspension 10 mg/ml

Ingredients:

Hypromellose powder   10 g

Purified Water, USP   **QSAD:** 1000 ml

Preparation Details:

1. Weigh out Hypromellose powder and add to a beaker.
2. Add one third of the water into the beaker and heat to 90°C with vigorous stirring until agglomerates disappear and particles are thoroughly wetted.
3. Add cold water (5°C) to volume and continue stirring until mixture is homogenous.
4. Allow solution to cool in icy water until thoroughly hydrated, then allow it to gradually warm to ambient temperature.
5. Autoclave at 121°C for 20 minutes.
6. Allow solution to cool to room temperature. Initial pH of gelatin solution should be approximately 4.

Storage Conditions: Room Temperature or Refrigerate

Study Container Type: Unknown

Expiration Date: 21 days

References

1. Helin-Tanninen M, Naaranlahti T, Kontra K, et al. Enteral suspension of nifedipine for neonates. Part 2. Stability of an extemporaneously compounded nifedipine suspension. *J Clin Pharm Ther.* 2001;26:59–66.

Isradipine Syrup 1 mg/ml

Ingredients:

Isradipine 5-mg capsule	24 capsules
Glycerin USP	Small amount
Simple Syrup NF	**QSAD:** 120 ml

Preparation Details:

1. Open capsules and empty contents into a mortar.
2. Triturate contents to a fine powder.
3. Levigate with a small amount of Glycerin to form a paste.
4. Add base solution in increasing amounts while mixing thoroughly.
5. Transfer contents of the mortar to a graduated cylinder.
6. Rinse the mortar and pestle with base solution and pour into graduated cylinder.
7. Add base solution to the graduated cylinder to achieve the total volume indicated above.
8. Transfer contents of the graduated cylinder into an appropriate size amber bottle.
9. Shake well to mix.

Storage Conditions: Refrigerate

Special Instructions: Shake well before use.

Study Container Type: Glass

Expiration Date: 35 days

References

1. MacDonald JL, Johnson CE, Jacobson P. Stability of isradipine in an extemporaneously compounded oral liquid. *Am J Hosp Pharm.* 1994;51:2409–2411.

Ketoconazole Suspension 20 mg/ml

Ingredients:

Ketoconazole 200-mg tablet	12 tablets
Ora-Sweet/Ora-Plus*	**QSAD:** 120 ml

Preparation Details:

1. Triturate tablets to a fine powder in a mortar and pestle.
2. Levigate with a small amount of base solution to form a paste.
3. Add base solution in increasing amounts while mixing thoroughly.
4. Transfer contents of the mortar to a graduated cylinder.
5. Rinse the mortar and pestle with base solution and pour into graduated cylinder.
6. Add base solution to the graduated cylinder to achieve the total volume indicated above.
7. Transfer contents of the graduated cylinder into an appropriate size amber bottle.
8. Shake well to mix.

Storage Conditions: Room Temperature or Refrigerate

Special Instructions: *Mix 60 ml of Ora-Sweet with 60 ml of Ora-Plus. Use mixture as base solution. Shake well before use.

Alternatives: May substitute base solution with cherry syrup or 60 ml of Ora-Sweet SF mixed with 60 ml of Ora-Plus.

Study Container Type: Plastic

Expiration Date: 60 days

References

1. Allen Jr LV, Erickson III MA. Stability of ketoconazole, metolazone, metronidazole, procainamide hydrochloride, and spironolactone in extemporaneously compounded oral liquids. *Am J Health-Syst Pharm.* 1996;53:2073–2078.

Labetalol Suspension 40 mg/ml

Ingredients:

Labetalol 300-mg tablet   16 tablets

Ora-Sweet/Ora-Plus*   **QSAD:** 120 ml

Preparation Details:

1. Triturate tablets to a fine powder in a mortar and pestle.
2. Levigate with a small amount of base solution to form a paste.
3. Add base solution in increasing amounts while mixing thoroughly.
4. Transfer contents of the mortar to a graduated cylinder.
5. Rinse the mortar and pestle with base solution and pour into graduated cylinder.
6. Add base solution to the graduated cylinder to achieve the total volume indicated above.
7. Transfer contents of the graduated cylinder into an appropriate size amber bottle.
8. Shake well to mix.

Storage Conditions: Room Temperature or Refrigerate

Special Instructions: *Mix 60 ml of Ora-Sweet with 60 ml of Ora-Plus. Use mixture as base solution. Shake well before use.

Alternatives: May substitute base solution with cherry syrup or 60 ml of Ora-Sweet SF mixed with 60 ml of Ora-Plus.

Study Container Type: Plastic

Expiration Date: 60 days

References

1. Allen Jr LV, Erickson III MA. Stability of labetalol hydrochloride, metoprolol tartrate, verapamil hydrochloride, and spironolactone with hydrochlorothiazide in extemporaneously compounded oral liquids. *Am J Health-Syst Pharm.* 1996;53:2304–2309.

Labetalol Syrup 10 mg/ml

Ingredients:

Labetalol 300-mg tablet   4 tablets

Simple Syrup NF   **QSAD:** 120 ml

Preparation Details:

1. Triturate tablets to a fine powder in a mortar and pestle.
2. Levigate with a small amount of base solution to form a paste.
3. Add base solution in increasing amounts while mixing thoroughly.
4. Transfer contents of the mortar to a graduated cylinder.
5. Rinse the mortar and pestle with base solution and pour into graduated cylinder.
6. Add base solution to the graduated cylinder to achieve the total volume indicated above.
7. Transfer contents of the graduated cylinder into an appropriate size amber bottle.
8. Filter solution through a coarse filter and then a 0.45-micron filter.
9. Shake well to mix.

Storage Conditions: Room Temperature or Refrigerate

Special Instructions: Shake well before use.

Alternatives: May substitute base solution with distilled water, apple juice, grape juice, or orange juice.

Study Container Type: Glass and plastic

Expiration Date: 28 days

References

1. Nahata MC. Stability of labetalol hydrochloride in distilled water, simple syrup, and three fruit juices. *DICP Ann Pharmacother.* 1991;25:465–469.

Lamotrigine Suspension 1 mg/ml

Ingredients:

Lamotrigine 100-mg tablet	1 tablet
Glycerin USP	Small amount
Ora-Sweet/Ora-Plus*	**QSAD:** 100 ml

Preparation Details:

1. Triturate tablet to a fine powder in a mortar and pestle.
2. Levigate with a small amount of Glycerin to form a paste.
3. Add base solution in increasing amounts while mixing thoroughly.
4. Transfer contents of the mortar to a graduated cylinder.
5. Rinse the mortar and pestle with base solution and pour into graduated cylinder.
6. Add base solution to the graduated cylinder to achieve the total volume indicated above.
7. Transfer contents of the graduated cylinder into an appropriate size amber bottle.
8. Shake well to mix.

Storage Conditions: Room Temperature or Refrigerate

Special Instructions: *Mix 50 ml of Ora-Sweet with 50 ml of Ora-Plus. Use mixture as base solution. Shake well before use.

Alternatives: May substitute base solution with 50 ml of Ora-Sweet SF mixed with 50 ml of Ora-Plus.

Study Container Type: Plastic

Expiration Date: 90 days

References

1. Nahata MC, Morosco RS, Hipple TF. Stability of lamotrigine in two extemporaneously prepared oral suspensions at 4 and 25°C. *Am J Health-Syst Pharm.* 1999;56:240–242.

Lansoprazole Solution 3 mg/ml

Ingredients:

Lansoprazole 30-mg capsule   12 capsules

Sodium Bicarbonate 8.4%   **QSAD:** 120 ml

Preparation Details:

1. Open capsules and empty contents into a mortar.
2. Add base solution to the beaker to achieve the total volume indicated above.
3. Place the beaker on a magnetic stirrer and stir for 30 minutes.
4. Transfer solution into an appropriate size amber bottle.
5. Shake well to mix.

Storage Conditions: Refrigerate

Special Instructions: Shake well before use.

Study Container Type: Plastic oral syringe

Expiration Date: 14 days

References

1. DiGiacinto JL, Olsen KM, Bergman KL, et al. Stability of suspension formulations of lansoprazole and omeprazole stored in amber-colored plastic oral syringes. *Ann Pharmacother.* 2000;34:600–605.

Levodopa 5 mg/ml and Carbidopa 1.25 mg/ml Suspension

Ingredients:

Levodopa 100 mg/Carbidopa 25-mg tablet   6 tablets

Ora-Sweet/Ora-Plus*   **QSAD:** 120 ml

Preparation Details:

1. Triturate tablets to a fine powder in a mortar and pestle.
2. Levigate with a small amount of base solution to form a paste.
3. Add base solution in increasing amounts while mixing thoroughly.
4. Transfer contents of the mortar to a graduated cylinder.
5. Rinse the mortar and pestle with base solution and pour into graduated cylinder.
6. Add base solution to the graduated cylinder to achieve the total volume indicated above.
7. Transfer contents of the graduated cylinder into an appropriate size amber bottle.
8. Shake well to mix.

Storage Conditions: Refrigerate

Special Instructions: *Mix 60 ml of Ora-Sweet with 60 ml of Ora-Plus. Use mixture as base solution. Expiration date of 28 days when stored at room temperature. Shake well before use.

Study Container Type: Plastic

Expiration Date: 42 days

References

1. Nahata MC, Morosco RS, Leguire LE. Development of two stable oral suspensions of levodopa-carbidopa for children with amblyopia. *J Pediatr Ophthal Strasb.* 2000;37:333–377.

Levothyroxine Solution 25 mcg/ml

Ingredients:

Levothyroxine 0.1-mg tablet	30 tablets
Glycerol	48 ml
Sterile Water for Irrigation	**QSAD:** 120 ml

Preparation Details:

1. Triturate tablets to a fine powder in a mortar and pestle.
2. Levigate with 48 ml of Glycerol to form paste.
3. Add base solution in increasing amounts while mixing thoroughly.
4. Transfer contents of the mortar to a graduated cylinder.
5. Rinse the mortar and pestle with base solution and pour into graduated cylinder.
6. Add base solution to the graduated cylinder to achieve the total volume indicated above.
7. Transfer contents of the graduated cylinder into an appropriate size amber bottle.
8. Shake well to mix.

Storage Conditions: Refrigerate

Special Instructions: Shake well before use.

Study Container Type: Plastic

Expiration Date: 8 days

References

1. Boulton DW, Fawcett P, Woods DJ. Stability of an extemporaneously compounded levothyroxine sodium oral liquid. *Am J Health-Syst Pharm.* 1996;53:1157–1161.

Lisinopril Suspension 1 mg/ml—Formulation 1

Ingredients:

Lisinopril 10-mg tablet   12 tablets

Ora-Sweet/Ora-Plus*   **QSAD:** 120 ml

Preparation Details:

1. Triturate tablets to a fine powder in a mortar and pestle.
2. Levigate with a small amount of base solution to form a paste.
3. Add base solution in increasing amounts while mixing thoroughly.
4. Transfer contents of the mortar to a graduated cylinder.
5. Rinse the mortar and pestle with base solution and pour into graduated cylinder.
6. Add base solution to the graduated cylinder to achieve the total volume indicated above.
7. Transfer contents of the graduated cylinder into an appropriate size amber bottle.
8. Shake well to mix.

Storage Conditions: Room Temperature or Refrigerate

Special Instructions: Shake well before use.

Alternatives: May substitute base solution with 111 ml Simple Syrup NF mixed with 9 ml Methylcellulose 1% (see page 60 for preparation directions) with expiration of 91 days refrigerated or 56 days at room temperature.

Study Container Type: Plastic

Expiration Date: 91 days

References

1. Nahata MC, Morosco RS. Stability of lisinopril in two liquid dosage forms. *Ann Pharmacother.* 2004;38:396–399.

Lisinopril Syrup 1 mg/ml—Formulation 2

Ingredients:

Lisinopril 10-mg tablet	12 tablets
Sodium Citrate 100 mg/ml and Citric Acid 66.8 mg/ml	18 ml
Purified Water USP	6 ml
Ora-Sweet SF	**QSAD:** 120 ml

Preparation Details:

1. Place tablets in an appropriate size amber bottle.
2. Add Purified Water in amber bottle and shake bottle for 1 minute.
3. Add Bictra in amber bottle and shake bottle again.
4. Add 96 ml Ora-Sweet NF and shake well to disperse contents.

Storage Conditions: Room Temperature

Special Instructions: Shake well before use.

Study Container Type: Plastic

Expiration Date: 28 days

References

1. Thompson KC, Zhao Z, Mazakas JM, et al. Characterization of an extemporaneous liquid formulation of lisinopril. *Am J Health-Syst Pharm.* 2003;60:69–74.

Lisinopril Syrup 2 mg/ml

Ingredients:

Lisinopril 5-mg tablet	48 tablets
Sterile Water for Irrigation	7 ml
Simple Syrup NF	**QSAD:** 120 ml

Preparation Details:

1. Triturate tablets to a fine powder in a mortar and pestle.
2. Levigate with Sterile Water for Irrigation to form a paste.
3. Add base solution in increasing amounts while mixing thoroughly.
4. Transfer contents of the mortar to a graduated cylinder.
5. Rinse the mortar and pestle with base solution and pour into graduated cylinder.
6. Add base solution to the graduated cylinder to achieve the total volume indicated above.
7. Transfer contents of the graduated cylinder into an appropriate size amber bottle.
8. Shake well to mix.

Storage Conditions: Room Temperature or Refrigerate

Special Instructions: Shake well before use.

Study Container Type: Plastic

Expiration Date: 30 days

References

1. Webster AA, English BA, Rose D. The stability of lisinopril as an extemporaneous syrup. *Int J Pharm Compound.* 1997;1:352–353.

Losartan Suspension 2.5 mg/ml

Ingredients:

Losartan 50-mg tablet	6 tablets
Purified Water USP	6 ml
Ora-Plus/Ora-Sweet SF*	**QSAD:** 120 ml

Preparation Details:

1. Place tablets in an appropriate size amber bottle.
2. Add Purified Water in amber bottle and shake bottle for 2 minutes.
3. Let solution stand for 1 hour and then shake for 1 minute to disperse the tablet contents.
4. Add 114 ml base solution and shake well for 1 minute to disperse contents.

Storage Conditions: Refrigerate

Special Instructions: *Mix 60 ml of Ora-Sweet SF with 60 ml of Ora-Plus. Use mixture as base solution. Shake well before use.

Study Container Type: Plastic

Expiration Date: 28 days

References

1. Cozaar® [package insert]. Whitehouse Station, NJ: Merck & Co; June 2009.

Mercaptopurine Syrup 50 mg/ml

Ingredients:

Mercaptopurine 50-mg tablet	100 tablets
Ascorbic Acid 100-mg tablet	1 tablet
Simple Syrup	33 ml
Sterile Water for Irrigation	17 ml
Cherry Syrup	**QSAD**: 100 ml

Preparation Details:

Must be prepared in a vertical hood. Must wear mask during preparation.

1. Triturate tablets to a fine powder in a mortar and pestle.
2. Levigate with Sterile Water for Irrigation to form a paste.
3. Add Simple Syrup in increasing amounts while mixing thoroughly.
4. Transfer contents of the mortar to a graduated cylinder.
5. Rinse the mortar and pestle with base solution and pour into graduated cylinder.
6. Add base solution to the graduated cylinder to achieve the total volume indicated above.
7. Transfer the solution into an appropriate size amber bottle.
8. Shake well to mix.

Storage Conditions: Room Temperature

Special Instructions: Shake well before use.

Alternatives: Syrup may be made without Ascorbic Acid with an expiration date of 35 days when stored in room temperature.

Study Container Type: Glass

Expiration Date: 77 days

References

1. Aliabadi HM, Romanick M, Desai S, et al. Effect of buffer and antioxidant on stability of a mercaptopurine suspension. *Am J Health-Syst Pharm.* 2008;65:441–448.

Methylcellulose Suspension 10 mg/ml

Ingredients:

Methylcellulose powder 4000 centipoises	10 g
Methylparaben powder	200 mg
Propylparaben powder	100 mg
Purified Water, USP	**QSAD:** 1000 ml

Preparation Details:

1. Heat 200 ml of Purified Water to boiling.
2. Add parabens in and mix well.
3. Wet the Methylcellulose powder and add to the hot solution.
4. Allow to stand for 15 minutes.
5. Remove from heat and qs with cold Purified Water while mixing well with a magnetic stirrer. Keep mixing until a clear, homogeneous solution results.

Storage Conditions: Room Temperature

Special Instructions: Shake well before use.

Study Container Type: Unknown

Expiration Date: 180 days

References

1. Nahata MC, Pai VB, Hipple TF. *Pediatric Drug Formulations*. 5th ed. Cincinnati, OH: Harvey Whitney Book Company; 2004.

Methyldopa Syrup 50 mg/ml

Ingredients:

Methyldopa 250-mg tablet	24 tablets
Simple Syrup NF	**QSAD:** 120 ml

Preparation Details:

1. Remove film coating off tablets with a wet paper towel.
2. Triturate tablets to a fine powder in a mortar and pestle.
3. Levigate with a small amount of base solution to form a paste.
4. Add base solution in increasing amounts while mixing thoroughly.
5. Transfer contents of the mortar to a graduated cylinder.
6. Rinse the mortar and pestle with base solution and pour into graduated cylinder.
7. Add base solution to the graduated cylinder to achieve the total volume indicated above.
8. Transfer contents of the graduated cylinder into an appropriate size amber bottle.
9. Shake well to mix.

Storage Conditions: Room Temperature or Refrigerate

Special Instructions: Shake well before use.

Study Container Type: Glass

Expiration Date: 14 days

References

1. Newton DW, Rogers AG, Becker CH, et al. Extemporaneous preparation of methyldopa in two syrup vehicles. *Am J Hosp Pharm.* 1975;32:817–821.

Metolazone Suspension 1 mg/ml

Ingredients:

Metolazone 10-mg tablet   12 tablets

Ora-Sweet/Ora-Plus*   **QSAD:** 120 ml

Preparation Details:

1. Triturate tablets to a fine powder in a mortar and pestle.
2. Levigate with a small amount of base solution to form a paste.
3. Add base solution in increasing amounts while mixing thoroughly.
4. Transfer contents of the mortar to a graduated cylinder.
5. Rinse the mortar and pestle with base solution and pour into graduated cylinder.
6. Add base solution to the graduated cylinder to achieve the total volume indicated above.
7. Transfer contents of the graduated cylinder into an appropriate size amber bottle.
8. Shake well to mix.

Storage Conditions: Room Temperature or Refrigerate

Special Instructions: *Mix 60 ml of Ora-Sweet with 60 ml of Ora-Plus. Use mixture as base solution. Shake well before use.

Alternatives: May substitute base solution with cherry syrup or 60 ml of Ora-Sweet SF mixed with 60 ml of Ora-Plus.

Study Container Type: Plastic

Expiration Date: 60 days

References

1. Allen Jr LV, Erickson III MA. Stability of ketoconazole, metolazone, metronidazole, procainamide hydrochloride, and spironolactone in extemporaneously compounded oral liquids. *Am J Health-Syst Pharm.* 1996;53:2073–2078.

Metoprolol Tartrate Suspension 10 mg/ml

Ingredients:

Metoprolol 100-mg tablet	12 tablets
Ora-Sweet/Ora-Plus*	**QSAD:** 120 ml

Preparation Details:

1. Triturate tablets to a fine powder in a mortar and pestle.
2. Levigate with a small amount of base solution to form a paste.
3. Add base solution in increasing amounts while mixing thoroughly.
4. Transfer contents of the mortar to a graduated cylinder.
5. Rinse the mortar and pestle with base solution and pour into graduated cylinder.
6. Add base solution to the graduated cylinder to achieve the total volume indicated above.
7. Transfer contents of the graduated cylinder into an appropriate size amber bottle.
8. Shake well to mix.

Storage Conditions: Room Temperature or Refrigerate

Special Instructions: *Mix 60 ml of Ora-Sweet with 60 ml of Ora-Plus. Use mixture as base solution. Shake well before use.

Alternatives: May substitute base solution with cherry syrup or 60 ml of Ora-Sweet SF mixed with 60 ml of Ora-Plus.

Study Container Type: Plastic

Expiration Date: 60 days

References

1. Allen Jr LV, Erickson III MA. Stability of labetalol hydrochloride, metoprolol tartrate, verapamil hydrochloride, and spironolactone with hydrochlorothiazide in extemporaneously compounded oral liquids. *Am J Health-Syst Pharm.* 1996;53:2304–2309.

Metronidazole Suspension 10 mg/ml

Ingredients:

Metronidazole 250-mg tablet   5 tablets

Ora-Sweet/Ora-Plus*   **QSAD:** 125 ml

Preparation Details:

1. Triturate tablets to a fine powder in a mortar and pestle.
2. Levigate with a small amount of glycerin to form a paste.
3. Add base solution in increasing amounts while mixing thoroughly.
4. Transfer contents of the mortar to a graduated cylinder.
5. Rinse the mortar and pestle with base solution and pour into graduated cylinder.
6. Add base solution to the graduated cylinder to achieve the total volume indicated above.
7. Transfer contents of the graduated cylinder into an appropriate size amber bottle.
8. Shake well to mix.

Storage Conditions: Room Temperature

Special Instructions: *Mix 62.5 ml of Ora-Sweet with 62.5 ml of Ora-Plus. Use mixture as base solution. Shake well before use.

Alternatives: May substitute base solution with Ora-Plus alone.

Study Container Type: Glass

Expiration Date: 90 days

References

1. Mathew M, Das Gupta V, Bethea C. Stability of metronidazole in solutions and suspensions. *J Clin Pharm Therapeutics.* 1994;19:27–29.

Metronidazole Suspension 50 mg/ml

Ingredients:

Metronidazole 250-mg tablet	24 tablets
Ora-Sweet/Ora-Plus*	**QSAD:** 120 ml

Preparation Details:

1. Triturate tablets to a fine powder in a mortar and pestle.
2. Levigate with a small amount of base solution to form a paste.
3. Add base solution in increasing amounts while mixing thoroughly.
4. Transfer contents of the mortar to a graduated cylinder.
5. Rinse the mortar and pestle with base solution and pour into graduated cylinder.
6. Add base solution to the graduated cylinder to achieve the total volume indicated above.
7. Transfer contents of the graduated cylinder into an appropriate size amber bottle.
8. Shake well to mix.

Storage Conditions: Room Temperature or Refrigerate

Special Instructions: *Mix 60 ml of Ora-Sweet with 60 ml of Ora-Plus. Use mixture as base solution. Shake well before use.

Alternatives: May substitute base solution with cherry syrup or 60 ml of Ora-Sweet SF mixed with 60 ml of Ora-Plus.

Study Container Type: Plastic

Expiration Date: 60 days

References

1. Allen Jr LV, Erickson III MA. Stability of ketoconazole, metolazone, metronidazole, procainamide hydrochloride, and spironolactone in extemporaneously compounded oral liquids. *Am J Health-Syst Pharm.* 1996;53:2073–2078.

Metronidazole Syrup 5 mg/ml

Ingredients:

Metronidazole 250-mg tablet	2 tablets
Ora-Sweet	**QSAD:** 100 ml

Preparation Details:

1. Triturate tablets to a fine powder in a mortar and pestle.
2. Levigate with a small amount of base solution to form a paste.
3. Add base solution in increasing amounts while mixing thoroughly.
4. Transfer contents of the mortar to a graduated cylinder.
5. Rinse the mortar and pestle with base solution and pour into graduated cylinder.
6. Add base solution to the graduated cylinder to achieve the total volume indicated above.
7. Transfer contents of the graduated cylinder into an appropriate size amber bottle.
8. Shake well to mix.

Storage Conditions: Room Temperature

Special Instructions: Shake well before use.

Study Container Type: Glass

Expiration Date: 90 days

References

1. Mathew M, Das Gupta V, Bethea C. Stability of metronidazole in solutions and suspensions. *J Clin Pharm Therapeutics.* 1994;19:27–29.

Mexiletine Solution 10 mg/ml

Ingredients:

Mexiletine 150-mg capsule	8 capsules
Sterile Water for Irrigation	**QSAD:** 120 ml

Preparation Details:

1. Open capsules and empty contents into a mortar.
2. Triturate contents to a fine powder.
3. Levigate with a small amount of base solution to form a paste.
4. Add base solution in increasing amounts while mixing thoroughly.
5. Transfer contents of the mortar to a graduated cylinder.
6. Rinse the mortar and pestle with base solution and pour into graduated cylinder.
7. Add base solution to the graduated cylinder to achieve the total volume indicated above.
8. Transfer contents of the graduated cylinder into an appropriate size amber bottle.
9. Shake well to mix.

Storage Conditions: Refrigerate

Special Instructions: Expiration date of 70 days at room temperature. Shake well before use.

Alternatives: May substitute base solution with sorbitol with an expiration date of 28 days under refrigeration and 14 days at room temperature.

Study Container Type: Plastic

Expiration Date: 91 days

References

1. Nahata MC, Morosco RS, Hipple TF. Stability of mexiletine in two extemporaneous liquid formulations stored under refrigeration and at room temperature. *J Am Pharm Assoc.* 2000;40:257–259.

Moxifloxacin Suspension 20 mg/ml

Ingredients:

Moxifloxacin 400-mg tablet   6 tablets

Ora-Sweet/Ora-Plus*   **QSAD:** 120 ml

Preparation Details:

1. Triturate tablets to a fine powder in a mortar and pestle.
2. Levigate with a small amount of base solution to form a paste.
3. Add base solution in increasing amounts while mixing thoroughly.
4. Transfer contents of the mortar to a graduated cylinder.
5. Rinse the mortar and pestle with base solution and pour into graduated cylinder.
6. Add base solution to the graduated cylinder to achieve the total volume indicated above.
7. Transfer contents of the graduated cylinder into an appropriate size amber bottle.
8. Shake well to mix.

Storage Conditions: Room Temperature

Special Instructions: *Mix 60 ml of Ora-Sweet with 60 ml of Ora-Plus. Use mixture as base solution. Shake well before use.

Alternatives: May substitute base solution with 60 ml of Ora-Sweet SF mixed with 60 ml of Ora-Plus.

Footnote: Strong, bitter aftertaste. Administer with masking agent, such as chocolate syrup or peanut butter, before and after medication administration.

Study Container Type: Plastic

Expiration Date: 90 days

References

1. Hutchinson DJ, Johnson CE, Klein KC. Stability of extemporaneously prepared moxifloxacin oral suspensions. *Am J Health-Syst Pharm.* 2009;66:665–667.

Naratriptan Suspension 0.5 mg/ml

Ingredients:

Naratriptan 2.5-mg tablet	24 tablets
Ora-Sweet/Ora-Plus*	**QSAD:** 120 ml

Preparation Details:

1. Triturate tablets to a fine powder in a mortar and pestle.
2. Levigate with a small amount of base solution to form a paste.
3. Add base solution in increasing amounts while mixing thoroughly.
4. Transfer contents of the mortar to a graduated cylinder.
5. Rinse the mortar and pestle with base solution and pour into graduated cylinder.
6. Add base solution to the graduated cylinder to achieve the total volume indicated above.
7. Transfer contents of the graduated cylinder into an appropriate size amber bottle.
8. Shake well to mix.

Storage Conditions: Refrigerate

Special Instructions: *Mix 60 ml of Ora-Sweet with 60 ml of Ora-Plus. Use mixture as base solution. Expiration date of 7 days when stored at room temperature. Shake well before use.

Alternatives: May substitute base solution with 60 ml of Ora-Sweet SF mixed with 60 ml of Ora-Plus.

Study Container Type: Plastic

Expiration Date: 90 days

References

1. Zhang YP, Trissel LA, Fox JL. Naratriptan hydrochloride in extemporaneously compounded oral suspensions. *Int J Pharm Compound.* 2000;4:69–71.

Nifedipine Solution 10 mg/ml

Ingredients:

Nifedipine powder	3.2 g
Glycerin USP	127 ml
Peppermint Oil	3.2 ml
Polyethylene Glycol 400	190 ml
	QSAD: 320 ml

Preparation Details:

1. Measure Polyethylene Glycol 400 and add to a beaker.
2. Weigh Nifedipine powder and add to Polyethylene Glycol 400 while stirring.
3. Measure Glycerin and add to Polyethylene Glycol 400 and Nifedipine while stirring.
4. Heat the cloudy, yellow liquid to approximately 95°C while stirring and maintain that temperature until all the Nifedipine dissolves.
5. Filter the hot, clear solution through a 1.2-micron glass microfiber filter and stir until the liquid cools to room temperature.
6. Add Peppermint Oil and pour the solution into an amber glass bottle.

Storage Conditions: Room Temperature, Protect from Light

Special Instructions: Expiration date of 14 days when stored in amber oral syringes.

Study Container Type: Glass

Expiration Date: 35 days

References

1. Dentinger PJ, Swenson CF, Anaizi NH. Stability of nifedipine in an extemporaneously compounded oral solution. *Am J Health-Syst Pharm.* 2003;60:1019–1022.

Nifedipine Suspension 1 mg/ml

Ingredients:

Nifedipine powder   120 mg

Hypromellose 1%   **QSAD:** 120 ml

Preparation Details:

See page 46 for preparation directions of Hypromellose 1%.
Suspensions should be prepared in a dimly lit room to prevent
photodegradation of Nifedipine.

1. Weigh out Nifedipine powder and add to mortar.
2. Levigate with a small amount of base solution to form a paste.
3. Add base solution in increasing amounts while mixing thoroughly.
4. Transfer contents of the mortar to a graduated cylinder.
5. Rinse the mortar and pestle with base solution and pour into graduated cylinder.
6. Add base solution to the graduated cylinder to achieve the total volume indicated above.
7. Transfer contents of the graduated cylinder into an appropriate size amber bottle.
8. Shake well to mix.

Storage Conditions: Room Temperature or Refrigerate, Protect from Light

Special Instructions: Shake well before use.

Study Container Type: Plastic syringe

Expiration Date: 21 days

References

1. Helin-Tanninen M, Naaranlahti T, Kontra K, et al. Enteral suspension of nifedipine for neonates. Part 2. Stability of an extemporaneously compounded nifedipine suspension. *J Clin Pharm Ther.* 2001;26:59–66.

Norfloxacin Suspension 20 mg/ml

Ingredients:

Norfloxacin 400-mg tablet	6 tablets
Strawberry Syrup/Ora-Plus*	**QSAD:** 120 ml

Preparation Details:

1. Triturate tablets to a fine powder in a mortar and pestle.
2. Levigate with a small amount of base solution to form a paste.
3. Add base solution in increasing amounts while mixing thoroughly.
4. Transfer contents of the mortar to a graduated cylinder.
5. Rinse the mortar and pestle with base solution and pour into graduated cylinder.
6. Add base solution to the graduated cylinder to achieve the total volume indicated above.
7. Transfer contents of the graduated cylinder into an appropriate size amber bottle.
8. Shake well to mix.

Storage Conditions: Room Temperature or Refrigerate

Special Instructions: *Mix 60 ml of Strawberry Syrup with 60 ml of Ora-Plus. Use mixture as base solution. Strawberry Syrup is prepared by mixing 160 ml of Simple Syrup NF and 30 ml of strawberry fountain syrup. Shake well before use.

Study Container Type: Plastic

Expiration Date: 56 days

References

1. Johnson CE, Price J, Hession JM. Stability of norfloxacin in an extemporaneously prepared oral liquid. *Am J Health-Syst Pharm.* 2001;58:577–579.

Omeprazole Solution 2 mg/ml

Ingredients:

Omeprazole 20-mg delayed release capsule   12 capsules

Sodium Bicarbonate 8.4%   **QSAD:**120 ml

Preparation Details:

1. Open capsules and empty contents into a mortar.
2. Add base solution to the beaker to achieve the total volume indicated above.
3. Place the beaker on a magnetic stirrer and stir for 30 minutes.
4. Transfer solution into an appropriate size amber bottle.
5. Shake well to mix.

Storage Conditions: Refrigerate

Special Instructions: Expiration date of 14 days at room temperature. Shake well before use.

Study Container Type: Amber-colored plastic syringe and glass

Expiration Date: 45 days

References

1. DiGiacinto JL, Olsen KM, Bergman KL, et al. Stability of suspension formulations of lansoprazole and omeprazole stored in amber-colored plastic oral syringes. *Ann Pharmacother.* 2000;34:600–604.

2. Quercia RA, Fan C, Liu X, et al. Stability of omeprazole in an extemporaneously prepared oral liquid. *Am J Health-Syst Pharm.* 1997;54:1833–1866.

Pantoprazole Solution 2 mg/ml—Formulation 1

Ingredients:

Pantoprazole 40-mg tablet	6 tablets
Sodium Bicarbonate powder	10.1 g
Sterile Water for Irrigation	**QSAD:** 120 ml

Preparation Details:

1. Remove imprint from tablets by gently rubbing on a paper towel dampened with ethanol.
2. Allow tablets to air dry for a few minutes.
3. Triturate tablets to a fine powder in a mortar and pestle.
4. Transfer the contents of the mortar to an appropriate size beaker.
5. Add 100 ml of Sterile Water for Irrigation and place the beaker on a magnetic stirrer.
6. Add 5 g of Sodium Bicarbonate powder and continue to stir for approximately 20 minutes until all tablet remnants have disintegrated and the coating has dissolved.
7. Add remaining Sodium Bicarbonate powder and stir for approximately 5 minutes until the powder dissolves.
8. Add enough Sterile Water for Irrigation to achieve the final volume indicated.
9. Transfer the solution into an appropriate size amber bottle.
10. Shake well to mix.

Storage Conditions: Refrigerate

Special Instructions: Shake well before use.

Study Container Type: Plastic

Expiration Date: 62 days

References

1. Dentinger PJ, Swenson CF, Anaizi NH. Stability of pantoprazole in an extemporaneously compounded oral liquid. *Am J Health-Syst Pharm.* 2002;59:953–956.

Pantoprazole Solution 2 mg/ml—Formulation 2

Ingredients:

Pantoprazole 40-mg tablet	6 tablets
Sodium Bicarbonate 4.2%	**QSAD:** 120 ml

Preparation Details:

1. Remove imprint from tablets by gently rubbing on a paper towel dampened with ethanol.
2. Allow tablets to air dry for a few minutes.
3. Triturate tablets to a fine powder in a mortar and pestle.
4. Transfer the contents of the mortar to an appropriate size beaker.
5. Add base solution to the beaker to achieve the total volume indicated above.
6. Place the beaker on a magnetic stirrer and stir for 30 minutes.
7. Transfer solution into an appropriate size amber bottle.
8. Shake well to mix.

Storage Conditions: Refrigerate

Special Instructions: Shake well before use.

Study Container Type: Plastic syringes

Expiration Date: 14 days

References

1. Ferron GM, Ku S, Abell M, et al. Oral bioavailability of pantoprazole suspended in sodium bicarbonate solution. *Am J Health-Syst Pharm.* 2003;60:1324–1329.

Pentoxifylline Solution 20 mg/ml

Ingredients:

Pentoxifylline 400-mg tablet	6 tablets
Sterile Water for Irrigation	**QSAD:** 120 ml

Preparation Details:

1. Triturate tablets to a fine powder in a mortar and pestle.
2. Levigate with a small amount of base solution to form a paste.
3. Add base solution in increasing amounts while mixing thoroughly.
4. Transfer contents of the mortar to a graduated cylinder.
5. Rinse the mortar and pestle with base solution and pour into graduated cylinder.
6. Add base solution to the graduated cylinder to achieve the total volume indicated above.
7. Transfer contents of the graduated cylinder into an appropriate size amber bottle.
8. Shake well to mix.

Storage Conditions: Room Temperature or Refrigerate

Special Instructions: Shake well before use.

Study Container Type: Glass and plastic

Expiration Date: 90 days

References

1. Abdel-Rahman SM, Nahata MC. Stability of pentoxifylline in an extemporaneously prepared oral suspension. *Am J Health-Syst Pharm.* 1997;54:1301–1303.

Phenoxybenzamine Solution 2 mg/ml

Ingredients:

Phenoxybenzamine 10-mg capsule	6 capsules
Citric Acid powder	45 mg
Propylene Glycol	0.3 ml
Sterile Water for Irrigation	**QSAD:** 30 ml

Preparation Details:

1. Open capsules and empty contents into a mortar.
2. Triturate contents to a fine powder.
3. Weigh out Citric Acid powder and add to mortar.
4. Measure and add Propylene Glycol to the powder in the mortar.
5. Levigate with a small amount of base solution to form a paste.
6. Add base solution in increasing amounts while mixing thoroughly.
7. Transfer contents of the mortar to a graduated cylinder.
8. Rinse the mortar and pestle with base solution and pour into graduated cylinder.
9. Add base solution to the graduated cylinder to achieve the total volume indicated above.
10. Transfer contents of the graduated cylinder into an appropriate size amber bottle.
11. Shake well to mix.

Storage Conditions: Refrigerate

Special Instructions: Shake well before use.

Study Container Type: Glass

Expiration Date: 7 days

References

1. Lim LY, Tan LL, Chan EWY, et al. Stability of phenoxybenzamine hydrochloride in various vehicles. *Am J Health-System Pharm.* 1997;54:2073–2078.

Potassium Perchlorate Solution 13.3 mg/ml

Ingredients:

Potassium Perchlorate 200-mg capsule	8 capsules
Sterile Water for Irrigation	**QSAD:** 120 ml

Preparation Details:

Must be prepared in a vertical hood. Must wear mask during preparation.

1. Open capsules and empty contents into a mortar.
2. Triturate contents to a fine powder.
3. Levigate with a small amount of base solution to form a paste.
4. Add base solution in increasing amounts while mixing thoroughly.
5. Transfer contents of the mortar to a graduated cylinder.
6. Rinse the mortar and pestle with base solution and pour into graduated cylinder.
7. Add base solution to the graduated cylinder to achieve the total volume indicated above.
8. Draw up the solution from the graduated cylinder into two 60-ml syringes.
9. Change to a 0.22-micron filter needle.
10. Filter solution into a 4-ounce glass bottle.

Storage Conditions: Room Temperature

Special Instructions: Shake well before use. Caution oxidizing agent.

Study Container Type: Glass

Expiration Date: 270 days

References

1. Williams CC. Stability of aqueous perchlorate formulations. *Am J Hosp Pharm.* 1977;34:93–95.

Propylthiouracil Suspension 5 mg/ml

Ingredients:

Propylthiouracil 50-mg tablet   12 tablets

Ora-Sweet/Ora-Plus*   **QSAD:** 120 ml

Preparation Details:

1. Triturate tablets to a fine powder in a mortar and pestle.
2. Levigate with a small amount of base solution to form a paste.
3. Add base solution in increasing amounts while mixing thoroughly.
4. Transfer contents of the mortar to a graduated cylinder.
5. Rinse the mortar and pestle with base solution and pour into graduated cylinder.
6. Add base solution to the graduated cylinder to achieve the total volume indicated above.
7. Transfer contents of the graduated cylinder into an appropriate size amber bottle.
8. Shake well to mix.

Storage Conditions: Refrigerate

Special Instructions: *Mix 60 ml of Ora-Sweet with 60 ml of Ora-Plus. Use mixture as base solution. Expiration date of 70 days when stored at room temperature. Shake well before use.

Alternatives: May substitute base solution with 60 ml Methylcellulose 1% (see page 60 for preparation directions) mixed with 60 ml Simple Syrup NF.

Study Container Type: Plastic

Expiration Date: 91 days

References

1. Nahata MC, Morosco RS, Trowbridge JM. Stability of propylthiouracil in extemporaneously prepared oral suspensions at 4 and 25°C. *Am J Health-Syst Pharm.* 2000;57:1141–1143.

Pyrazinamide Suspension 10 mg/ml

Ingredients:

Pyrazinamide 500-mg tablet   3 tablets

Ora-Sweet/Ora-Plus*   **QSAD:** 150 ml

Preparation Details:

1. Triturate tablets to a fine powder in a mortar and pestle.
2. Levigate with a small amount of base solution to form a paste.
3. Add base solution in increasing amounts while mixing thoroughly.
4. Transfer contents of the mortar to a graduated cylinder.
5. Rinse the mortar and pestle with base solution and pour into graduated cylinder.
6. Add base solution to the graduated cylinder to achieve the total volume indicated above.
7. Transfer contents of the graduated cylinder into an appropriate size amber bottle.
8. Shake well to mix.

Storage Conditions: Room Temperature or Refrigerate

Special Instructions: *Mix 75 ml of Ora-Sweet with 75 ml of Ora-Plus. Use mixture as base solution. Shake well before use.

Alternatives: May substitute base solution with cherry syrup or 75 ml of Ora-Sweet SF mixed with 75 ml of Ora-Plus.

Study Container Type: Plastic

Expiration Date: 60 days

References

1. Allen Jr LV, Erickson III MA. Stability of bethanechol chloride, pyrazinamide, quinidine sulfate, rifampin, and tetracycline hydrochloride in extemporaneously compounded oral liquids. *Am J Health-Syst Pharm.* 1998;55:1804–1809.

Pyrazinamide Syrup 100 mg/ml

Ingredients:

Pyrazinamide 500-mg tablet	24 tablets
Simple Syrup	**QSAD:** 120 ml

Preparation Details:

1. Triturate tablets to a fine powder in a mortar and pestle.
2. Levigate with a small amount of base solution to form a paste.
3. Add base solution in increasing amounts while mixing thoroughly.
4. Transfer contents of the mortar to a graduated cylinder.
5. Rinse the mortar and pestle with base solution and pour into graduated cylinder.
6. Add base solution to the graduated cylinder to achieve the total volume indicated above.
7. Transfer contents of the graduated cylinder into an appropriate size amber bottle.
8. Shake well to mix.

Storage Conditions: Room Temperature or Refrigerate

Special Instructions: Shake well before use.

Alternatives: May substitute base solution with 60 ml Methylcellulose 1% (see page 60 for preparation directions) mixed with 60 ml Simple Syrup NF.

Study Container Type: Glass and plastic

Expiration Date: 60 days

References

1. Nahata MC, Morosco RS, Peritore SP. Stability of pyrazinamide in two suspensions. *Am J Health-Syst Pharm.* 1995;52:1558–1560.

Pyrimethamine Suspension 2 mg/ml

Ingredients:

Pyrimethamine 25-mg tablet	10 tablets
Simple Syrup/Methylcellulose 1%*	**QSAD:** 125 ml

Preparation Details:

1. Triturate tablets to a fine powder in a mortar and pestle.
2. Levigate with a small amount of base solution to form a paste.
3. Add base solution in increasing amounts while mixing thoroughly.
4. Transfer contents of the mortar to a graduated cylinder.
5. Rinse the mortar and pestle with base solution and pour into graduated cylinder.
6. Add base solution to the graduated cylinder to achieve the total volume indicated above.
7. Transfer contents of the graduated cylinder into an appropriate size amber bottle.
8. Shake well to mix.

Storage Conditions: Room Temperature or Refrigerate

Special Instructions: *Mix 62.5 ml of Simple Syrup with 62.5 ml of Methylcellulose 1% (see page 60 for preparation directions). Use mixture as base solution. Shake well before use.

Study Container Type: Glass and plastic

Expiration Date: 91 days

References

1. Nahata MC, Morosco RS, Hipple TF. Stability of pyrimethamine in a liquid dosage formulation stored for three months. *Am J Health-Syst Pharm.* 1997;54:2714–2716.

Quinidine Sulfate Suspension 10 mg/ml

Ingredients:

Quinidine 200-mg tablet   6 tablets

Ora-Sweet/Ora-Plus*   **QSAD:** 120 ml

Preparation Details:

1. Triturate tablets to a fine powder in a mortar and pestle.
2. Levigate with a small amount of base solution to form a paste.
3. Add base solution in increasing amounts while mixing thoroughly.
4. Transfer contents of the mortar to a graduated cylinder.
5. Rinse the mortar and pestle with base solution and pour into graduated cylinder.
6. Add base solution to the graduated cylinder to achieve the total volume indicated above.
7. Transfer contents of the graduated cylinder into an appropriate size amber bottle.
8. Shake well to mix.

Storage Conditions: Room Temperature or Refrigerate

Special Instructions: *Mix 60 ml of Ora-Sweet with 60 ml of Ora-Plus. Use mixture as base solution. Shake well before use.

Alternatives: May substitute base solution with cherry syrup or 60 ml of Ora-Sweet SF mixed with 60 ml of Ora-Plus.

Study Container Type: Plastic

Expiration Date: 60 days

References

1. Allen Jr LV, Erickson III MA. Stability of bethanechol chloride, pyrazinamide, quinidine sulfate, rifampin, and tetracycline hydrochloride in extemporaneously compounded oral liquids. *Am J Health-Syst Pharm.* 1998;55:1804–1809.

Rifabutin Suspension 20 mg/ml

Ingredients:

Rifabutin 150-mg capsule	16 capsules
Ora-Sweet/Ora-Plus*	**QSAD:** 120 ml

Preparation Details:

1. Open capsules and empty contents into a mortar.
2. Triturate contents to a fine powder.
3. Levigate with a small amount of base solution to form a paste.
4. Add base solution in increasing amounts while mixing thoroughly.
5. Transfer contents of the mortar to a graduated cylinder.
6. Rinse the mortar and pestle with base solution and pour into graduated cylinder.
7. Add base solution to the graduated cylinder to achieve the total volume indicated above.
8. Transfer contents of the graduated cylinder into an appropriate size amber bottle.
9. Shake well to mix.

Storage Conditions: Room Temperature or Refrigerate

Special Instructions: *Mix 60 ml of Ora-Sweet with 60 ml of Ora-Plus. Use mixture as base solution. Shake well before use.

Alternatives: May substitute base solution with cherry syrup.

Study Container Type: Plastic

Expiration Date: 84 days

References

1. Haslam JL, Egodage KL, Chen Y, et al. Stability of rifabutin in two extemporaneously compounded oral liquids. *Am J Health-Syst Pharm.* 1999;56:333–336.

Rifampin Suspension 25 mg/ml

Ingredients:

Rifampin 300-mg capsule   10 capsules

Ora-Sweet/Ora-Plus*   **QSAD:** 120 ml

Preparation Details:

1. Open capsules and empty contents into a mortar.
2. Triturate contents to a fine powder.
3. Levigate with a small amount of base solution to form a paste.
4. Add base solution in increasing amounts while mixing thoroughly.
5. Transfer contents of the mortar to a graduated cylinder.
6. Rinse the mortar and pestle with base solution and pour into graduated cylinder.
7. Add base solution to the graduated cylinder to achieve the total volume indicated above.
8. Transfer contents of the graduated cylinder into an appropriate size amber bottle.
9. Shake well to mix.

Storage Conditions: Room Temperature or Refrigerate

Special Instructions: *Mix 60 ml of Ora-Sweet with 60 ml of Ora-Plus. Use mixture as base solution. Shake well before use.

Alternatives: May substitute base solution with cherry syrup or 60 ml of Ora-Sweet SF mixed with 60 ml of Ora-Plus.

Study Container Type: Plastic

Expiration Date: 28 days

References

1. Allen Jr LV, Erickson III MA. Stability of bethanechol chloride, pyrazinamide, quinidine sulfate, rifampin, and tetracycline hydrochloride in extemporaneously compounded oral liquids. *Am J Health-Syst Pharm.* 1998;55:1804–1809.

Rifampin Syrup 10 mg/ml

Ingredients:

Rifampin 600-mg injection vial	2 vials
Sterile Water for Injection	20 ml
Simple Syrup	**QSAD:** 120 ml

Preparation Details:

1. Reconstitute each vial of injectable powder with 10 ml of Sterile Water for Injection.
2. Withdraw the contents from each vial into a syringe.
3. Transfer the solution to a graduated cylinder.
4. Add base solution to the graduated cylinder to achieve the total volume indicated above.
5. Transfer contents of the graduated cylinder into an appropriate size amber bottle.
6. Shake well to mix.

Storage Conditions: Room Temperature or Refrigerate

Special Instructions: Shake well before use.

Footnote: Syrup prepared from capsules may be nonhomogeneous and lead to unpredictable dosing.

Study Container Type: Plastic

Expiration Date: 56 days

References

1. Nahata MC, Morosco RS, Hipple TF. Stability of rifampin in two suspensions at room temperature. *J Clin Pharm Ther.* 1994;19:263–265.

2. Nahata MC, Morosco RS, Hipple TF. Effect of preparation method and storage on rifampin concentration in suspensions. *Ann Pharmacother.* 1994;28:182–185.

Sildenafil Suspension 2.5 mg/ml

Incredients:

Sildenafil 100-mg tablet   3 tablets

Ora-Sweet/Ora-Plus*   **QSAD:** 120 ml

Preparation Details:

1. Triturate tablets to a fine powder in a mortar and pestle.
2. Levigate with a small amount of base solution to form a paste.
3. Add base solution in increasing amounts while mixing thoroughly.
4. Transfer contents of the mortar to a graduated cylinder.
5. Rinse the mortar and pestle with base solution and pour into graduated cylinder.
6. Add base solution to the graduated cylinder to achieve the total volume indicated above.
7. Transfer contents of the graduated cylinder into an appropriate size amber bottle.
8. Shake well to mix.

Storage Conditions: Room Temperature or Refrigerate

Special Instructions: *Mix 60 ml of Ora-Plus with 60 ml of Ora-Sweet. Use mixture as base solution. Shake well before use.

Alternatives: May substitute base solution with 60 ml Methylcellulose 1% (see page 60 for preparation directions) mixed with 60 ml Simple Syrup NF.

Study Container Type: Plastic

Expiration Date: 91 days

References

1. Nahata MC, Morosco RS, Brady MT. Extemporaneous sildenafil citrate oral suspensions for the treatment of pulmonary hypertension in children. *Am J Health-Syst Pharm*. 2006;63:254–257.

Sotalol Suspension 5 mg/ml

Ingredients:

Sotalol 120-mg tablet	5 tablets
Ora-Sweet/Ora-Plus*	**QSAD:** 120 ml

Preparation Details:

1. Triturate tablets to a fine powder in a mortar and pestle.
2. Levigate with a small amount of base solution to form a paste.
3. Add base solution in increasing amounts while mixing thoroughly.
4. Transfer contents of the mortar to a graduated cylinder.
5. Rinse the mortar and pestle with base solution and pour into graduated cylinder.
6. Add base solution to the graduated cylinder to achieve the total volume indicated above.
7. Transfer contents of the graduated cylinder into an appropriate size amber bottle.
8. Shake well to mix.

Storage Conditions: Room Temperature or Refrigerate

Special Instructions: *Mix 60 ml of Ora-Plus with 60 ml of Ora-Sweet. Use mixture as base solution. Shake well before use.

Alternatives: *May substitute base solution with 108 ml Simple Syrup NF mixed with 12 ml Methylcellulose 1% (see page 60 for preparation directions).

Study Container Type: Plastic

Expiration Date: 90 days

References

1. Nahata MC, Morosco RS. Stability of sotalol in two liquid formulations at two temperatures. *Ann Pharmacother.* 2003;l37:506–509.

Spironolactone 5 mg/ml and Hydrochlorothiazide 5 mg/ml

Ingredients:

Spironolactone 25-mg/Hydrochlorothiazide
25-mg tablet

24 tablets

Ora-Sweet/Ora-Plus*

QSAD: 120 ml

Preparation Details:

1. Triturate tablets to a fine powder in a mortar and pestle.
2. Levigate with a small amount of base solution to form a paste.
3. Add base solution in increasing amounts while mixing thoroughly.
4. Transfer contents of the mortar to a graduated cylinder.
5. Rinse the mortar and pestle with base solution and pour into graduated cylinder.
6. Add base solution to the graduated cylinder to achieve the total volume indicated above.
7. Transfer contents of the graduated cylinder into an appropriate size amber bottle.
8. Shake well to mix.

Storage Conditions: Room Temperature or Refrigerate

Special Instructions: *Mix 60 ml of Ora-Sweet with 60 ml of Ora-Plus. Use mixture as base solution. Shake well before use.

Alternatives: May substitute base solution with cherry syrup or 60 ml of Ora-Sweet SF mixed with 60 ml of Ora-Plus.

Study Container Type: Plastic

Expiration Date: 60 days

References

1. Allen Jr LV, Erickson III MA. Stability of labetalol hydrochloride, metoprolol tartrate, verapamil hydrochloride, and spironolactone with hydrochlorothiazide in extemporaneously compounded oral liquids. *Am J Health-Syst Pharm.* 1996;53:2304–2309.

Spironolactone Suspension 25 mg/ml

Ingredients:

Spironolactone 25-mg tablet	120 tablets
Ora-Sweet/Ora-Plus*	**QSAD:** 120 ml

Preparation Details:

1. Triturate tablets to a fine powder in a mortar and pestle.
2. Levigate with a small amount of base solution to form a paste.
3. Add base solution in increasing amounts while mixing thoroughly.
4. Transfer contents of the mortar to a graduated cylinder.
5. Rinse the mortar and pestle with base solution and pour into graduated cylinder.
6. Add base solution to the graduated cylinder to achieve the total volume indicated above.
7. Transfer contents of the graduated cylinder into an appropriate size amber bottle.
8. Shake well to mix.

Storage Conditions: Room Temperature or Refrigerate

Special Instructions: *Mix 60 ml of Ora-Sweet with 60 ml of Ora-Plus. Use mixture as base solution. Shake well before use.

Alternatives: May substitute base solution with cherry syrup or 60 ml of Ora-Sweet SF mixed with 60 ml of Ora-Plus.

Study Container Type: Plastic

Expiration Date: 60 days

References

1. Allen Jr LV, Erickson III MA. Stability of ketoconazole, metolazone, metronidazole, procainamide hydrochloride, and spironolactone in extemporaneously compounded oral liquids. *Am J Health-Syst Pharm.* 1996;53:2073–2078.

Spironolactone Syrup 2.5 mg/ml

Ingredients:

Spironolactone 25-mg tablet	12 tablets
Purified Water USP	5 ml
Cherry Syrup	**QSAD:** 120 ml

Preparation Details:

1. Triturate tablets to a fine powder in a mortar and pestle.
2. Levigate with 5 ml of Purified Water USP to form a paste.
3. Add base solution in increasing amounts while mixing thoroughly.
4. Transfer contents of the mortar to a graduated cylinder.
5. Rinse the mortar and pestle with base solution and pour into graduated cylinder.
6. Add base solution to the graduated cylinder to achieve the total volume indicated above.
7. Transfer contents of the graduated cylinder into an appropriate size amber bottle.
8. Shake well to mix.

Storage Conditions: Room Temperature or Refrigerate

Special Instructions: Shake well before use.

Study Container Type: Glass

Expiration Date: 28 days

References

1. Mathur LK, Wickman A. Stability of extemporaneously compounded spironolactone suspensions. *Am J Hosp Pharm.* 1989;46:2040–2042.

Spironolactone Syrup 5 mg/ml

Ingredients:

Spironolactone 50-mg tablet	12 tablets
Purified Water USP	5 ml
Cherry Syrup	**QSAD:** 120 ml

Preparation Details:

1. Triturate tablets to a fine powder in a mortar and pestle.
2. Levigate with 5 ml of Purified Water USP to form a paste.
3. Add base solution in increasing amounts while mixing thoroughly.
4. Transfer contents of the mortar to a graduated cylinder.
5. Rinse the mortar and pestle with base solution and pour into graduated cylinder.
6. Add base solution to the graduated cylinder to achieve the total volume indicated above.
7. Transfer contents of the graduated cylinder into an appropriate size amber bottle.
8. Shake well to mix.

Storage Conditions: Room Temperature or Refrigerate

Special Instructions: Shake well before use.

Study Container Type: Glass

Expiration Date: 28 days

References

1. Mathur LK, Wickman A. Stability of extemporaneously compounded spironolactone suspensions. *Am J Hosp Pharm.* 1989;46:2040–2042.

Spironolactone Syrup 10 mg/ml

Ingredients:

Spironolactone 100-mg tablet   12 tablets

Purified Water USP   5 ml

Cherry Syrup   **QSAD:** 120 ml

Preparation Details:

1. Triturate tablets to a fine powder in a mortar and pestle.
2. Levigate with 5 ml of Purified Water USP to form a paste.
3. Add base solution in increasing amounts while mixing thoroughly.
4. Transfer contents of the mortar to a graduated cylinder.
5. Rinse the mortar and pestle with base solution and pour into graduated cylinder.
6. Add base solution to the graduated cylinder to achieve the total volume indicated above.
7. Transfer contents of the graduated cylinder into an appropriate size amber bottle.
8. Shake well to mix.

Storage Conditions: Room Temperature or Refrigerate

Special Instructions: Shake well before use.

Study Container Type: Glass

Expiration Date: 28 days

References

1. Mathur LK, Wickman A. Stability of extemporaneously compounded spironolactone suspensions. *Am J Hosp Pharm.* 1989;46:2040–2042.

Sulfasalazine Suspension 100 mg/ml

Ingredients:

Sulfasalazine 500-mg tablet	24 tablets
Ora-Sweet/Ora-Plus*	**QSAD:** 120 ml

Preparation Details:

1. Triturate tablets to a fine powder in a mortar and pestle.
2. Levigate with a small amount of base solution to form a paste.
3. Add base solution in increasing amounts while mixing thoroughly.
4. Transfer contents of the mortar to a graduated cylinder.
5. Rinse the mortar and pestle with base solution and pour into graduated cylinder.
6. Add base solution to the graduated cylinder to achieve the total volume indicated above.
7. Transfer contents of the graduated cylinder into an appropriate size amber bottle.
8. Shake well to mix.

Storage Conditions: Room Temperature or Refrigerate

Special Instructions: Do not use enteric-coated tablets. Shake well before use.

Study Container Type: Glass and plastic

Expiration Date: 91 days

References

1. Lingertat-Walsh K, Walker SE, Law S, et al. Stability of sulfasalazine oral suspension. *Can J Hosp Pharm.* 2006;59:194–200.

Sumatriptan Suspension 5 mg/ml

Ingredients:

Sumatriptan 100-mg tablet	6 tablets
Ora-Plus	30 ml
Ora-Sweet	**QSAD:** 120 ml

Preparation Details:

1. Triturate tablets to a fine powder in a mortar and pestle.
2. Levigate with 30 ml of Ora-Plus to form paste.
3. Add base solution in increasing amounts while mixing thoroughly.
4. Transfer contents of the mortar to a graduated cylinder.
5. Rinse the mortar and pestle with base solution and pour into graduated cylinder.
6. Add base solution to the graduated cylinder to achieve the total volume indicated above.
7. Transfer contents of the graduated cylinder into an appropriate size amber bottle.
8. Shake well to mix.

Storage Conditions: Refrigerate

Special Instructions: Shake well before use.

Alternatives: May substitute base solution with Ora-Sweet SF or Syrpalta. It is not necessary to use Ora-Plus if Syrpalta is used as base.

Study Container Type: Glass

Expiration Date: 21 days

References

1. Fish DN, Beall HD, Goodwin SD, et al. Stability of sumatriptan succinate in extemporaneously prepared oral liquids. *Am J Health-Syst Pharm.* 1997;54:1619–1622.

Tacrolimus Suspension 0.5 mg/ml

Ingredients:

Tacrolimus 5-mg capsule	12 capsules
Simple Syrup/Ora-Plus*	**QSAD:** 120 ml

Preparation Details:

1. Open capsules and empty contents into a mortar.
2. Triturate contents to a fine powder.
3. Levigate with a small amount of base solution to form a paste.
4. Add base solution in increasing amounts while mixing thoroughly.
5. Transfer contents of the mortar to a graduated cylinder.
6. Rinse the mortar and pestle with base solution and pour into graduated cylinder.
7. Add base solution to the graduated cylinder to achieve the total volume indicated above.
8. Transfer contents of the graduated cylinder into an appropriate size amber bottle.
9. Shake well to mix.

Storage Conditions: Room Temperature

Special Instructions: *Mix 60 ml of Simple Syrup with 60 ml of Ora-Plus. Use mixture as base solution. Shake well before use.

Study Container Type: Glass and plastic

Expiration Date: 56 days

References

1. Jacobson PA, Johnson CE, West NJ, et al. Stability of tacrolimus in an extemporaneously compounded oral liquid. *Am J Health-Syst Pharm.* 1997;54:178–180.

Tacrolimus Suspension 1 mg/ml

Ingredients:

Tacrolimus 5-mg capsule   24 capsules

Ora-Sweet/Ora-Plus*   **QSAD:** 120 ml

Preparation Details:

1. Open capsules and empty contents into a mortar.
2. Triturate contents to a fine powder.
3. Levigate with a small amount of base solution to form a paste.
4. Add base solution in increasing amounts while mixing thoroughly.
5. Transfer contents of the mortar to a graduated cylinder.
6. Rinse the mortar and pestle with base solution and pour into graduated cylinder.
7. Add base solution to the graduated cylinder to achieve the total volume indicated above.
8. Transfer contents of the graduated cylinder into an appropriate size amber bottle.
9. Shake well to mix.

Storage Conditions: Room Temperature

Special Instructions: *Mix 60 ml of Ora-Sweet with 60 ml of Ora-Plus. Use mixture as base solution. Shake well before use.

Study Container Type: Plastic

Expiration Date: 120 days

References

1. Elefante A, Muindi J, West K, et al. Long-term stability of a patient-convenient 1 mg/ml suspension of tacrolimus for accurate maintenance of stable therapeutic levels. *Bone Marrow Transplant.* 2006;37:781–784.

Temozolomide Suspension 10 mg/ml

Ingredients:

Temozolomide 100-mg capsule	12 capsules
Anhydrous Citric Acid	30 mg
Povidone K-30 powder	600 mg
Purified Water USP	1.8 ml
Ora-Sweet/Ora-Plus*	**QSAD:** 120 ml

Preparation Details:

Must be prepared in a vertical hood. Must wear mask during preparation.

1. Open capsules and empty contents into a mortar.
2. Weigh Povidone K-30 powder and place in mortar.
3. Triturate contents to a fine powder.
4. Dissolve Anhydrous Citric Acid in Purified Water USP.
5. Levigate powder with mixture of Anhydrous Citric Acid and Purified Water to form a paste.
6. Add base solution in increasing amounts while mixing thoroughly.
7. Transfer contents of the mortar to a graduated cylinder.
8. Rinse the mortar and pestle with base solution and pour into graduated cylinder.
9. Add base solution to the graduated cylinder to achieve the total volume indicated above.
10. Transfer contents of the graduated cylinder into an appropriate size amber bottle.
11. Shake well to mix.

Storage Conditions: Refrigerate

Special Instructions: *Mix 60 ml of Ora-Sweet with 60 ml of Ora-Plus. Use mixture as base solution. Shake well before use.

Alternatives: May substitute base solution with 60 ml of Ora-Plus mixed with 60 ml of Ora-Sweet SF.

Study Container Type: Plastic

Expiration Date: 60 days

References

1. Trissel LA, Zhang Y, Koontz SE. Temozolomide stability in extemporaneously compounded oral suspension. *Int J Pharm Compound.* 2006;10:396–399.

Terbinafine Suspension 25 mg/ml

Ingredients:

Terbinafine 250-mg tablet	12 tablets
Ora-Sweet/Ora-Plus*	**QSAD:** 120 ml

Preparation Details:

1. Triturate tablets to a fine powder in a mortar and pestle.
2. Levigate with a small amount of base solution to form a paste.
3. Add base solution in increasing amounts while mixing thoroughly.
4. Transfer contents of the mortar to a graduated cylinder.
5. Rinse the mortar and pestle with base solution and pour into graduated cylinder.
6. Add base solution to the graduated cylinder to achieve the total volume indicated above.
7. Transfer contents of the graduated cylinder into an appropriate size amber bottle.
8. Shake well to mix.

Storage Conditions: Room Temperature or Refrigerate

Special Instructions: *Mix 60 ml of Ora-Sweet with 60 ml of Ora-Plus. Use mixture as base solution. Shake well before use.

Study Container Type: Plastic

Expiration Date: 42 days

References

1. Abdel-Rahman SM, Nahata MC. Stability of terbinafine hydrochloride in an extemporaneously prepared oral suspension at 25 and 4°C. *Am J Health-Syst Pharm.* 1999;56:243–245.

Terbutaline Syrup 1 mg/ml

Ingredients:

Terbutaline 5-mg tablet	24 tablets
Purified Water USP	5 ml
Simple Syrup NF	**QSAD:** 120 ml

Preparation Details:

1. Triturate tablets to a fine powder in a mortar and pestle.
2. Levigate with Purified Water USP to form a paste.
3. Add base solution in increasing amounts while mixing thoroughly.
4. Transfer contents of the mortar to a graduated cylinder.
5. Rinse the mortar and pestle with base solution and pour into graduated cylinder.
6. Add base solution to the graduated cylinder to achieve the total volume indicated above.
7. Transfer contents of the graduated cylinder into an appropriate size amber bottle.
8. Shake well to mix.

Storage Conditions: Refrigerate

Special Instructions: Shake well before use.

Study Container Type: Glass

Expiration Date: 55 days

References

1. Horner RK, Johnson CE. Stability of an extemporaneously compounded terbutaline sulfate oral liquid. *Am J Hosp Pharm.* 1991;48:293–295.

Tetracycline Suspension 25 mg/ml

Ingredients:

Tetracycline 250-mg capsule	12 capsules
Ora-Sweet/Ora-Plus*	**QSAD:** 120 ml

Preparation Details:

1. Open capsules and empty contents into a mortar.
2. Triturate contents to a fine powder.
3. Levigate with a small amount of base solution to form a paste.
4. Add base solution in increasing amounts while mixing thoroughly.
5. Transfer contents of the mortar to a graduated cylinder.
6. Rinse the mortar and pestle with base solution and pour into graduated cylinder.
7. Add base solution to the graduated cylinder to achieve the total volume indicated above.
8. Transfer contents of the graduated cylinder into an appropriate size amber bottle.
9. Shake well to mix.

Storage Conditions: Room Temperature or Refrigerate

Special Instructions: *Mix 60 ml of Ora-Sweet with 60 ml of Ora-Plus. Use mixture as base solution. Shake well before use.

Alternatives: May substitute base solution with 60 ml of Ora-Plus mixed with 60 ml of Ora-Sweet SF with expiration date of 10 days refrigerated and 7 days when stored at room temperature.

Study Container Type: Plastic

Expiration Date: 28 days

References

1. Allen Jr LV, Erickson III MA. Stability of bethanechol chloride, pyrazinamide, quinidine sulfate, rifampin, and tetracycline hydrochloride in extemporaneously compounded oral liquids. *Am J Health-Syst Pharm.* 1998;55:1804–1809.

Tiagabine Suspension 1 mg/ml

Ingredients:

Tiagabine 12-mg tablet	10 tablets
Ora-Sweet/Ora-Plus*	**QSAD:** 120 ml

Preparation Details:

1. Triturate tablets to a fine powder in a mortar and pestle.
2. Levigate with a small amount of base solution to form a paste.
3. Add base solution in increasing amounts while mixing thoroughly.
4. Transfer contents of the mortar to a graduated cylinder.
5. Rinse the mortar and pestle with base solution and pour into graduated cylinder.
6. Add base solution to the graduated cylinder to achieve the total volume indicated above.
7. Transfer contents of the graduated cylinder into an appropriate size amber bottle.
8. Shake well to mix.

Storage Conditions: Refrigerate

Special Instructions: *Mix 60 ml of Ora-Plus with 60 ml of Ora-Sweet. Use mixture as base solution. Expiration date of 70 days when stored at room temperature. Shake well before use.

Alternatives: May substitute base solution with 17 ml Methylcellulose 1% (see page 60 for preparation directions) mixed with 103 ml Simple Syrup NF with an expiration date of 91 days refrigerated and 42 days when stored at room temperature.

Study Container Type: Plastic

Expiration Date: 91 days

References

1. Nahata MC, Morosco RS. Stability of tiagabine in two oral liquid vehicles. *Am J Health-Syst Pharm.* 2003;60:75–77.

Topiramate Suspension 6 mg/ml

Ingredients:

Topiramate 100-mg tablet   6 tablets

Ora-Sweet/Ora-Plus*   **QSAD:** 100 ml

Preparation Details:

1. Triturate tablets to a fine powder in a mortar and pestle.
2. Levigate with a small amount of base solution to form a paste.
3. Add base solution in increasing amounts while mixing thoroughly.
4. Transfer contents of the mortar to a graduated cylinder.
5. Rinse the mortar and pestle with base solution and pour into graduated cylinder.
6. Add base solution to the graduated cylinder to achieve the total volume indicated above.
7. Transfer contents of the graduated cylinder into an appropriate size amber bottle.
8. Shake well to mix.

Storage Conditions: Room Temperature or Refrigerate

Special Instructions: *Mix 50 ml of Ora-Plus with 50 ml of Ora-Sweet. Use mixture as base solution. Shake well before use.

Alternatives: May substitute base solution with 12.5 ml Methylcellulose 1% (see page 60 for preparation directions) mixed with 87.5 ml Simple Syrup NF.

Study Container Type: Plastic

Expiration Date: 28 days

References

1. Nahata MC, Morosco RS, Willhite EA. Topiramate stability in two oral suspensions stored in plastic prescription bottles at two temperatures. *IPA*. ASHP Midyear Meeting, 2001;36:P–77R.

Tramadol 7.5 mg/ml and Acetaminophen 65 mg/ml Suspension

Ingredients:

Tramadol 37.5-mg/Acetaminophen 325-mg tablet   24 tablets

Ora-Plus/Ora-Sweet SF*   **QSAD:** 120 ml

Preparation Details:

1. Triturate tablets to a fine powder in a mortar and pestle.
2. Levigate with a small amount of base solution to form a paste.
3. Add base solution in increasing amounts while mixing thoroughly.
4. Transfer contents of the mortar to a graduated cylinder.
5. Rinse the mortar and pestle with base solution and pour into graduated cylinder.
6. Add base solution to the graduated cylinder to achieve the total volume indicated above.
7. Transfer contents of the graduated cylinder into an appropriate size amber bottle.
8. Shake well to mix.

Storage Conditions: Room Temperature or Refrigerate

Special Instructions: *Mix 60 ml of Ora-Plus with 60 ml of Ora-Sweet SF. Use mixture as base solution. Shake well before use.

Alternatives: May substitute base solution with 60 ml of Ora-Plus mixed with 60 ml of strawberry syrup. Strawberry syrup is prepared by mixing 160 ml of Simple Syrup NF and 30 ml of strawberry fountain syrup.

Study Container Type: Plastic

Expiration Date: 90 days

References

1. Johnson CE, Wagner DS, DeLoach SL, et al. Stability of tramadol hydrochloride-acetaminophen (Ultracet) in strawberry syrup and in a sugar-free vehicle. *Am J Health-Syst Pharm.* 2004;61:54–57.

Tramadol Suspension 5 mg/ml

Ingredients:

Tramadol 50-mg tablet   12 tablets

Ora-Plus/Ora-Sweet SF*   **QSAD:** 120 ml

Preparation Details:

1. Triturate tablets to a fine powder in a mortar and pestle.
2. Levigate with a small amount of base solution to form a paste.
3. Add base solution in increasing amounts while mixing thoroughly.
4. Transfer contents of the mortar to a graduated cylinder.
5. Rinse the mortar and pestle with base solution and pour into graduated cylinder.
6. Add base solution to the graduated cylinder to achieve the total volume indicated above.
7. Transfer contents of the graduated cylinder into an appropriate size amber bottle.
8. Shake well to mix.

Storage Conditions: Room Temperature or Refrigerate

Special Instructions: *Mix 60 ml of Ora-Plus with 60 ml of Ora-Sweet SF. Use mixture as base solution. Shake well before use.

Alternatives: May substitute base solution with 60 ml of Ora-Plus mixed with 60 ml of strawberry syrup. Strawberry syrup is prepared by mixing 160 ml of Simple Syrup NF and 30 ml of strawberry fountain syrup.

Study Container Type: Plastic

Expiration Date: 90 days

References

1. Wagner DS, Johnson CE, Cichon-Hensley BK, et al. Stability of oral liquid preparations of tramadol in strawberry syrup and in a sugar-free vehicle. *Am J Health-Syst Pharm.* 2003;60:1268–1270.

Ursodiol Suspension 25 mg/ml

Ingredients:

Ursodiol 300-mg capsule	10 capsules
Glycerin USP	10 ml
Ora-Plus	60 ml
Orange Syrup NF	**QSAD:** 120 ml

Preparation Details:

1. Open capsules and empty contents into a mortar.
2. Triturate contents to a fine powder.
3. Levigate with Glycerin to form a paste.
4. Add Ora-Plus in increasing amounts while mixing thoroughly.
5. Transfer contents of the mortar to a graduated cylinder.
6. Rinse the mortar and pestle with base solution and pour into graduated cylinder.
7. Add base solution to the graduated cylinder to achieve the total volume indicated above.
8. Transfer contents of the graduated cylinder into an appropriate size amber bottle.
9. Shake well to mix.

Storage Conditions: Room Temperature or Refrigerate

Special Instructions: Shake well before use.

Study Container Type: Plastic

Expiration Date: 60 days

References

1. Mallett MS, Hagan RL, Peters DA. Stability of ursodiol 25 mg/ml in an extemporaneously prepared oral liquid. *Am J Health-Syst Pharm*. 1997;54:1401–1404.

Ursodiol Suspension 50 mg/ml

Ingredients:

Ursodiol 250-mg tablet	24 tablets
Ora-Plus/Ora-Sweet SF*	**QSAD:** 120 ml

Preparation Details:

1. Triturate tablets to a fine powder in a mortar and pestle.
2. Levigate with a small amount of base solution to form a paste.
3. Add base solution in increasing amounts while mixing thoroughly.
4. Transfer contents of the mortar to a graduated cylinder.
5. Rinse the mortar and pestle with base solution and pour into graduated cylinder.
6. Add base solution to the graduated cylinder to achieve the total volume indicated above.
7. Transfer contents of the graduated cylinder into an appropriate size amber bottle.
8. Shake well to mix.

Storage Conditions: Room Temperature or Refrigerate

Special Instructions: *Mix 60 ml of Ora-Sweet SF with 60 ml of Ora-Plus. Use mixture as base solution. Shake well before use.

Alternatives: May substitute base solution with 60 ml of strawberry syrup mixed with 60 ml of Ora-Plus. Strawberry syrup is prepared by mixing 160 ml of Simple Syrup NF and 30 ml of strawberry fountain syrup.

Study Container Type: Plastic

Expiration Date: 90 days

References

1. Johnson CE, Streetman DD. Stability of oral suspensions of ursodiol made from tablets. *Am J Health-Syst Pharm.* 2002;59:361–363.

Ursodiol Syrup 60 mg/ml

Ingredients:

Ursodiol 300-mg capsule	24 capsules
Glycerin USP	10 ml
Simple Syrup NF	**QSAD:** 120 ml

Preparation Details:

1. Open capsules and empty contents into a mortar.
2. Triturate contents to a fine powder.
3. Levigate with Glycerin to form a paste.
4. Add base solution in increasing amounts while mixing thoroughly.
5. Transfer contents of the mortar to a graduated cylinder.
6. Rinse the mortar and pestle with base solution and pour into graduated cylinder.
7. Add base solution to the graduated cylinder to achieve the total volume indicated above.
8. Transfer contents of the graduated cylinder into an appropriate size amber bottle.
9. Shake well to mix.

Storage Conditions: Refrigerate

Special Instructions: Shake well before use.

Study Container Type: Glass

Expiration Date: 35 days

References

1. Johnson CE, Nesbitt J. Stability of ursodiol in an extemporaneously compounded oral liquid. *Am J Health-Syst Pharm.* 1995;52:1798–1800.

Valacyclovir Suspension 50 mg/ml

Ingredients:

Valacyclovir 500-mg tablet	18 tablets
Ora-Plus	40 ml
Ora-Sweet	**QSAD:** 180 ml

Preparation Details:

1. Triturate tablets to a fine powder in a mortar and pestle.
2. Levigate with Ora-Plus to form paste.
3. Add base solution in increasing amounts while mixing thoroughly.
4. Transfer contents of the mortar to a graduated cylinder.
5. Rinse the mortar and pestle with base solution and pour into graduated cylinder.
6. Add base solution to the graduated cylinder to achieve the total volume indicated above.
7. Transfer contents of the graduated cylinder into an appropriate size amber bottle.
8. Shake well to mix.

Storage Conditions: Refrigerate

Special Instructions: Shake well before use.

Alternatives: May substitute base solution with Ora-Sweet SF or Syrpalta. It is not necessary to use Ora-Plus if Syrpalta is used as base solution. Suspension made from Syrpalta has an expiration date of 35 days under refrigeration.

Study Container Type: Glass

Expiration Date: 21 days

References

1. Fish DN, Vidaurri VA, Deeter RG. Stability of valacyclovir hydrochloride in extemporaneously prepared oral liquids. *Am J Heath-Syst Pharm.* 1999;56:1957–1960.

Verapamil Suspension 50 mg/ml

Ingredients:

Verapamil 80-mg tablet   75 tablets

Ora-Sweet/Ora-Plus*   **QSAD:** 120 ml

Preparation Details:

1. Triturate tablets to a fine powder in a mortar and pestle.
2. Levigate with a small amount of base solution to form a paste.
3. Add base solution in increasing amounts while mixing thoroughly.
4. Transfer contents of the mortar to a graduated cylinder.
5. Rinse the mortar and pestle with base solution and pour into graduated cylinder.
6. Add base solution to the graduated cylinder to achieve the total volume indicated above.
7. Transfer contents of the graduated cylinder into an appropriate size amber bottle.
8. Shake well to mix.

Storage Conditions: Room Temperature or Refrigerate

Special Instructions: *Mix 60 ml of Ora-Sweet with 60 ml of Ora-Plus. Use mixture as base solution. Shake well before use.

Alternatives: May substitute base solution with cherry syrup or 60 ml of Ora-Sweet SF mixed with 60 ml of Ora-Plus.

Study Container Type: Plastic

Expiration Date: 60 days

References

1. Allen Jr LV, Erickson III MA. Stability of labetalol hydrochloride, metoprolol tartrate, verapamil hydrochloride, and spironolactone with hydrochlorothiazide in extemporaneously compounded oral liquids. *Am J Health-Syst Pharm.* 1996;53:2304–2309.

Zonisamide Syrup 10 mg/ml

Ingredients:

Zonisamide 100-mg capsule   12 capsules

Simple Syrup NF   **QSAD:** 120 ml

Preparation Details:

1. Open capsules and empty contents into a mortar.
2. Triturate contents to a fine powder.
3. Levigate with a small amount of base solution to form a paste.
4. Add base solution in increasing amounts while mixing thoroughly.
5. Transfer contents of the mortar to a graduated cylinder.
6. Rinse the mortar and pestle with base solution and pour into graduated cylinder.
7. Add base solution to the graduated cylinder to achieve the total volume indicated above.
8. Transfer contents of the graduated cylinder into an appropriate size amber bottle.
9. Shake well to mix.

Storage Conditions: Room Temperature or Refrigerate

Special Instructions: Shake well before use.

Study Container Type: Plastic

Expiration Date: 28 days

References

1. Abobo CV, Wei B, Liang D. Stability of zonisamide in extemporaneously compounded oral suspensions. *Am J Health-Syst Pharm.* 2009;66:1105–1109.

Ointment/Ophthalmic Solution

Bacitracin Ophthalmic Solution 9,600 units/ml

Ingredients:

Bacitracin 50,000-units injection vial	3 vials
Artificial Tears	**QSAD:** 15.6 ml

Preparation Details:

Must be prepared in a laminar flow hood.

1. Reconstitute each vial of injectable powder with 3 ml of Artificial Tears from the 15-ml bottle.
2. Withdraw the contents from each vial into a syringe, total volume 9.6 ml.
3. Change to a 0.22-micron filter needle.
4. Transfer the reconstituted solution into the ophthalmic bottle with the remaining 6 ml Artificial Tears.
5. Shake well to mix.

Storage Conditions: Room Temperature

Special Instructions: Artificial Tears contains 0.5% hydroxypropyl methylcellulose. For ophthalmic use only.

Study Container Type: Plastic

Expiration Date: 7 days

References

1. Osborn E, Baum JL, Ernst C, et al. The stability of ten antibiotics in artificial tears solution. *Am J Ophthalmol.* 1976;82:775–780.

Cefazolin Ophthalmic Solution 33 mg/ml

Ingredients:

Cefazolin 500-mg injection vial	1 vial
Artificial Tears	**QSAD:** 15 ml

Preparation Details:

Must be prepared in a laminar flow hood.

1. Reconstitute injectable powder with 2 ml of Artificial Tears.
2. Withdraw volume of injectable solution using a 3-ml syringe.
3. Change to a 0.22-micron filter needle.
4. Transfer the reconstituted solution into a sterile, pyrogen-free ophthalmic dropper bottle.
5. Add base solution to the bottle to achieve the total volume indicated above.
6. Shake well to mix.

Storage Conditions: Refrigerate

Special Instructions: For ophthalmic use only.

Study Container Type: Plastic

Expiration Date: 28 days

References

1. Charlton JF, Dalla KP, Kniska A. Storage of extemporaneously prepared ophthalmic antimicrobial solutions. *Am J Health-Syst Pharm.* 1998;55:463–466.

Cidofovir Intravitreous Solution 0.2 mg/ml

Ingredients:

Cidofovir 75-mg/ml injection   0.13 ml

Sodium Chloride 0.9% injection   **QSAD:** 50 ml

Preparation Details:

Must be prepared in a laminar flow hood.

1. Withdraw volume of injectable solution using a 1-ml syringe.
2. Withdraw volume of base solution using a 60-ml syringe.
3. Add injectable solution into the syringe containing base solution.
4. Cap 60-ml syringe and mix well.
5. Change to a 0.22-micron filter needle.
6. Transfer the solution into an empty Viaflex bag.

Storage Conditions: Refrigerate

Special Instructions: For ophthalmic use only.

Study Container Type: Polyvinyl chloride or ethylene and propylene bags

Expiration Date: 5 days

References

1. Ennis RD, Dahl TC. Stability of cidofovir in 0.9% sodium chloride injection for five days. *Am J Health-Syst Pharm.* 1997;54:2204–2206.

Cidofovir Intravitreous Solution 8.1 mg/ml

Ingredients:

Cidofovir 75-mg/ml injection	5.4 ml
Sodium Chloride 0.9% injection	**QSAD:** 50 ml

Preparation Details:

Must be prepared in a laminar flow hood.

1. Withdraw volume of injectable solution using a 10-ml syringe.
2. Withdraw volume of base solution using a 60-ml syringe.
3. Add injectable solution into the syringe containing base solution.
4. Cap 60-ml syringe and mix well.
5. Change to a 0.22-micron filter needle.
6. Transfer the solution into an empty Viaflex bag.

Storage Conditions: Refrigerate

Special Instructions: For ophthalmic use only.

Study Container Type: Polyvinyl chloride or ethylene and propylene bags

Expiration Date: 5 days

References

1. Ennis RD, Dahl TC. Stability of cidofovir in 0.9% sodium chloride injection for five days. *Am J Health-Syst Pharm.* 1997;54:2204–2206.

Fumagillin Ophthalmic Solution 70 mcg/ml

Ingredients:

Fumagillin Bicyclohexylammonium crystals   120 mg

Sodium Chloride 0.9% for Injection   20 ml

Dacriose ophthalmic irrigating solution   **QSAD:** 40 ml

Preparation Details:

Must be prepared in a laminar flow hood.

1. Weigh out Fumagillin crystals and place them in an autoclaved beaker.
2. Add 10 ml of Sodium Chloride 0.9% for Injection to the beaker and mix to dissolve the crystals.
3. Withdraw the solution into a 60-ml syringe.
4. Rinse the beaker with 10 ml of Sodium Chloride 0.9% for Injection and withdraw the solution into the same 60-ml syringe.
5. Rinse the beaker with 20 ml of Dacriose ophthalmic irrigating solution and withdraw the solution into the same 60-ml syringe.
6. Cap 60-ml syringe and mix well.
7. Remove syringe cap and attach a 0.22-micron filter needle to the 60-ml syringe.
8. Transfer solution into a sterile, pyrogen-free ophthalmic dropper bottle.

Storage Conditions: Refrigerate and Protect from Light

Special Instructions: 3 mg/ml of Fumagillin Bicyclohexylammonium = 10 mg/ml of Fumagillin. For ophthalmic use only.

Study Container Type: Plastic

Expiration Date: 14 days

References

1. Abdel-Rahman SM, Nahata MC. Stability of fumagillin in an extemporaneously prepared ophthalmic solution. *Am J Health-Syst Pharm.* 1999;56:547–550.

Ganciclovir Intravitreous Solution 20 mg/ml

Ingredients:

Ganciclovir 500-mg injection vial	1 vial
Sterile Water for Injection	10 ml
Sodium Chloride 0.9% for Injection	**QSAD:** 25 ml

Preparation Details:

Must be prepared in a vertical hood. Must wear mask during preparation.

1. Reconstitute injectable powder with 10 ml of Sterile Water for Injection.
2. Withdraw volume of base solution using a 60-ml syringe.
3. Add injectable solution into the syringe-containing base solution.
4. Cap 60-ml syringe and mix well.
5. Change to a 0.22-micron filter needle.
6. Transfer the solution into a sterile vial.

Storage Conditions: Room Temperature or Refrigerate

Special Instructions: For ophthalmic use only. Caution teratogenic agent.

Study Container Type: Unknown

Expiration Date: 24 days

References

1. Morlet N, Young S, Naidoo D, et al. High dose intravitreal ganciclovir for CMV retinitis: a shelf life and cost comparison study. *Brit J Opth.* 1995;79:753–755.

Gentamicin Ophthalmic Solution 13.6 mg/ml (Fortified)

Ingredients:

Gentamicin 40-mg/ml injection   2 ml

Gentamicin opthalmic solution (3 mg/ml) **QSAD:** 7 ml

Preparation Details:

Must be prepared in a laminar flow hood.

1. Withdraw volume of injectable solution using a 3-ml syringe.
2. Change to a 0.22-micron filter needle.
3. Add injectable solution into the Gentamicin ophthalmic bottle.
4. Shake well to mix.

Storage Conditions: Refrigerate

Special Instructions: For ophthalmic use only.

Study Container Type: Plastic

Expiration Date: 90 days

References

1. McBride HA, Martinez DR, Trang JM, et al. Stability of gentamicin sulfate and tobramycin sulfate in extemporaneously prepared ophthalmic solutions at 8°C. *Am J Hosp Pharm.* 1991;48:507–509.

LET (Lidocaine 4%/Racepinephrine 0.225%/Tetracaine 0.5%) Solution

Ingredients:

Lidocaine 20% injection	10 ml
Racemic Epinephrine 2.25% inhalation solution	5 ml
Sodium Metabisulfite	31.5 mg
Tetracaine 2% injection	12.5 ml
Sterile Water for Injection	**QSAD:** 50 ml

Preparation Details:

Must be prepared in a laminar flow hood.

1. Measure out Lidocaine, Racepinephrine, Tetracaine, and Sterile Water for Injection into a beaker.
2. Weigh out Sodium Metabisulfite and add to the solution, mixing well.
3. Transfer the solution into an appropriate size amber bottle.

Storage Conditions: Refrigerate and Protect from Light

Special Instructions: Solution should have a blue tint. Expiration date of 28 days when stored at room temperature. For topical use only.

Study Container Type: Glass

Expiration Date: 182 days

References

1. Larson TA, Uden DL, Schilling CG. Stability of epinephrine hydrochloride in an extemporaneously compounded topical anesthetic solution of lidocaine, racepinephrine and tetracaine. *Am J Health-Syst Pharm.* 1996;53:659–662.

Tobramycin Ophthalmic Solution 13.6 mg/ml (Fortified)

Ingredients:

Tobramycin 40-mg/ml injection   2 ml

Tobramycin ophthalmic solution (3 mg/ml)   **QSAD:** 7 ml

Preparation Details:

Must be prepared in a laminar flow hood.

1. Withdraw volume of injectable solution using a 3-ml syringe.
2. Change to a 0.22-micron filter needle.
3. Add injectable solution into the Tobramycin ophthalmic bottle.
4. Shake well to mix.

Storage Conditions: Refrigerate

Special Instructions: For opthalmic use only.

Study Container Type: Plastic

Expiration Date: 90 days

References

1. McBride HA, Martinez DR, Trang JM, et al. Stability of gentamicin sulfate and tobramycin sulfate in extemporaneously prepared ophthalmic solutions at 8°C. *Am J Hosp Pharm.* 1991;48: 507–509.

Tobramycin Ophthalmic Solution 15 mg/ml

Ingredients:

Tobramycin 40-mg/ml injection	3.75 ml
Artificial Tears	**QSAD:** 10 ml

Preparation Details:

Must be prepared in a laminar flow hood.

1. Withdraw volume of injectable solution using a 5-ml syringe.
2. Change to a 0.22-micron filter needle.
3. Transfer solution into a sterile, pyrogen-free ophthalmic dropper bottle.
4. Add base solution to the bottle to achieve the total volume indicated above.
5. Shake well to mix.

Storage Conditions: Room Temperature or Refrigerate

Special Instructions: For ophthalmic use only.

Study Container Type: Plastic

Expiration Date: 28 days

References

1. Charlton JF, Dalla KP, Kniska A. Storage of extemporaneously prepared ophthalmic antimicrobial solutions. *Am J Health-Syst Pharm.* 1998;55:463–466.

Vancomycin Ophthalmic Solution 31 mg/ml

Ingredients:

Vancomycin 500-mg injection vial	1 vial
Sterile Water for Injection	5 ml
Artificial Tears	**QSAD:** 15 ml

Preparation Details:

Must be prepared in a laminar flow hood.

1. Reconstitute injectable powder with 5 ml of Sterile Water for Injection.
2. Withdraw 4.6 ml of Artificial Tears from the 15-ml ophthalmic bottle and discard.
3. Withdraw 4.6 ml of Vancomycin injectable solution using a 5-ml syringe.
4. Change to a 0.22-micron filter needle.
5. Transfer the Vancomycin solution into the ophthalmic bottle with the remaining Artificial Tears.
6. Shake well to mix.

Storage Conditions: Refrigerate

Special Instructions: For ophthalmic use only. Expiration date of 7 days when stored at room temperature.

Study Container Type: Plastic

Expiration Date: 10 days

References

1. Fuhrman Jr LC, Stroman RT. Stability of vancomycin in an extemporaneously compounded ophthalmic solution. *Am J Health-Syst Pharm.* 1998;55:1386–1388.

2. Osborn E, Baum JL, Ernst C, et al. The stability of ten antibiotics in artificial tear solutions. *Am J Ophthal.* 1976;82:775–780.

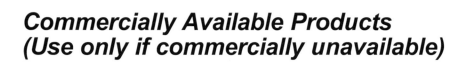

Commercially Available Products
(Use only if commercially unavailable)

Alprazolam Suspension 1 mg/ml

Ingredients:

Alprazolam 2-mg tablet	60 tablets
Ora-Sweet/Ora-Plus*	**QSAD:** 120 ml

Preparation Details:

1. Triturate tablets to a fine powder in a mortar and pestle.
2. Levigate with a small amount of base solution to form a paste.
3. Add base solution in increasing amounts while mixing thoroughly.
4. Transfer contents of the mortar to a graduated cylinder.
5. Rinse the mortar and pestle with base solution and pour into graduated cylinder.
6. Add base solution to the graduated cylinder to achieve the total volume indicated above.
7. Transfer contents of the graduated cylinder into an appropriate size amber bottle.
8. Shake well to mix.

Storage Conditions: Room Temperature or Refrigerate

Special Instructions: *Mix 60 ml of Ora-Sweet with 60 ml of Ora-Plus. Use mixture as base solution. Shake well before use.

Alternatives: May substitute base solution with cherry syrup or 60 ml of Ora-Sweet SF mixed with 60 ml of Ora-Plus.

Commercially Available: Use extemporaneously prepared formulation only when commercial product is unavailable.

Study Container Type: Plastic

Expiration Date: 60 days

References

1. Allen Jr LV, Erickson III MA. Stability of alprazolam, chloroquine phosphate, cisapride, enalapril maleate, and hydralazine hydrochloride in extemporaneously compounded oral liquids. *Am J Health-Syst Pharm.* 1998;55:1915–1920.

Caffeine Citrate Solution 10 mg/ml

Ingredients:

Caffeine Citrate powder	1.2 g
Citric Acid powder	1.2 g
Sterile Water for Irrigation	**QSAD:** 120 ml

Preparation Details:

1. Weigh out Caffeine Citrate and Citric Acid powder.
2. Dissolve in a graduated cylinder to the volume of Sterile Water for Irrigation indicated above.
3. Transfer the solution into an appropriate size amber bottle.
4. Shake well to mix.

Storage Conditions: Room Temperature

Special Instructions: Caffeine Citrate 10 mg/ml = Caffeine Base 5 mg/ml. Shake well before use.

Commercially Available (as a 20-mg/ml solution): Use extemporaneously prepared formulation only when commercial product is unavailable or a more dilute solution is desired.

Study Container Type: Glass

Expiration Date: 90 days

References

1. Hopkin C, Taylor A, Hanson S. Stability study of caffeine citrate. *Br J Pharm Practice.* 1990;4:122.

Caffeine Citrate Solution 20 mg/ml—Formulation 1

Ingredients:

Caffeine Citrate powder   9.6 g

Sterile Water for Irrigation   **QSAD:** 480 ml

Preparation Details:

1. Weigh out Caffeine Citrate powder.
2. Dissolve in a graduated cylinder to the volume of Sterile Water for Irrigation indicated above.
3. Transfer the solution into an appropriate size amber bottle.
4. Shake well to mix.

Storage Conditions: Room Temperature or Refrigerate

Special Instructions: Caffeine Citrate 20 mg/ml = Caffeine Base 10 mg/ml. Shake well before use.

Commercially Available: Use extemporaneously prepared formulation only when commercial product is unavailable.

Study Container Type: Glass

Expiration Date: 342 days

References

1. Donnelly RF, Tirona RG. Stability of citrated caffeine injectable solution in glass vials. *Am J Hosp Pharm.* 1994;51:512–514.

Caffeine Citrate Syrup 20 mg/ml—Formulation 2

Ingredients:

Caffeine Citrate powder	9.6 g
Sterile Water for Irrigation	240 ml
Cherry Syrup/Simple Syrup*	**QSAD:** 480 ml

Preparation Details:

1. Weigh out Caffeine Citrate powder.
2. Dissolve in a graduated cylinder to the volume of Sterile Water for Irrigation indicated above.
3. Add base solution to the graduated cylinder to achieve the total volume indicated above.
4. Transfer solution into an appropriate size amber bottle.
5. Shake well to mix.

Storage Conditions: Room Temperature

Special Instructions: *Mix 80 ml of Cherry Syrup with 160 ml of Simple Syrup. Use mixture as base solution. Caffeine Citrate 20 mg/ml = Caffeine Base 10 mg/ml. Shake well before use.

Commercially Available: Use extemporaneously prepared formulation only when commercial product is unavailable.

Study Container Type: Unknown

Expiration Date: 90 days

References

1. Eisenberg MG, Kang N. Stability of citrated caffeine solutions for injectable and enteral use. *Am J Hosp Pharm.* 1984;41:2405–2406.

Carbamazepine Syrup 40 mg/ml

Ingredients:

Carbamazepine 200-mg tablet   24 tablets

Simple Syrup   **QSAD:** 120 ml

Preparation Details:

1. Triturate tablets to a fine powder in a mortar and pestle.
2. Levigate with a small amount of base solution to form a paste.
3. Add base solution in increasing amounts while mixing thoroughly.
4. Transfer contents of the mortar to a graduated cylinder.
5. Rinse the mortar and pestle with base solution and pour into graduated cylinder.
6. Add base solution to the graduated cylinder to achieve the total volume indicated above.
7. Transfer contents of the graduated cylinder into an appropriate size amber bottle.
8. Shake well to mix.

Storage Conditions: Room Temperature or Refrigerate

Special Instructions: Shake well before use.

Commercially Available (as a 20-mg/ml suspension): Use extemporaneously prepared formulation only when commercial product is unavailable or a more concentrated syrup is desired.

Study Container Type: Glass

Expiration Date: 90 days

References

1. Burckart GJ, Hammond RW, Akers MJ. Stability of extemporaneous suspensions of carbamazepine. *Am J Hosp Pharm.* 1981;38:1929–1931.

Cimetidine Syrup 60 mg/ml

Ingredients:

Cimetidine 300-mg tablet	24 tablets
Glycerin USP	10 ml
Sterile Water for Irrigation	5 ml
Simple Syrup	**QSAD:** 120 ml

Preparation Details:

1. Allow tablets to stand in Sterile Water for 3–5 minutes to dissolve the film coating.
2. Triturate tablets to a fine powder in a mortar and pestle.
3. Levigate with a small amount of Glycerin to form a paste.
4. Add base solution in increasing amounts while mixing thoroughly.
5. Transfer contents of the mortar to a graduated cylinder.
6. Rinse the mortar and pestle with base solution and pour into graduated cylinder.
7. Add base solution to the graduated cylinder to achieve the total volume indicated above.
8. Transfer contents of the graduated cylinder into an appropriate size amber bottle.
9. Shake well to mix.

Storage Conditions: Refrigerate

Special Instructions: Shake well before use.

Commercially Available: Use extemporaneously prepared formulation only when commercial product is unavailable.

Study Container Type: Unknown

Expiration Date: 17 days

References

1. Tortorici MP. Formulation of a cimetidine oral suspension. *Am J Hosp Pharm.* 1979;36:22.

2. Sparkman HE. Experience with cimetidine oral suspension formulation. *Am J Hosp Pharm.* 1979;36: 600.

Ciprofloxacin Suspension 50 mg/ml

Ingredients:

Ciprofloxacin 250-mg tablet	24 tablets
Simple Syrup NF/Ora-Plus*	**QSAD:** 120 ml

Preparation Details:

1. Triturate tablets to a fine powder in a mortar and pestle.
2. Levigate with a small amount of base solution to form a paste.
3. Add base solution in increasing amounts while mixing thoroughly.
4. Transfer contents of the mortar to a graduated cylinder.
5. Rinse the mortar and pestle with base solution and pour into graduated cylinder.
6. Add base solution to the graduated cylinder to achieve the total volume indicated above.
7. Transfer contents of the graduated cylinder into an appropriate size amber bottle.
8. Shake well to mix.

Storage Conditions: Room Temperature or Refrigerate

Special Instructions: *Mix 60 ml of Simple Syrup NF with 60 ml of Ora-Plus. Use mixture as base solution. Shake well before use.

Commercially Available: Use extemporaneously prepared formulation only when commercial product is unavailable.

Study Container Type: Plastic

Expiration Date: 56 days

References

1. Johnson CE, Wong DV, Hoppe HL, et al. Stability of ciprofloxacin in an extemporaneous oral liquid dosage form. *Int J Pharm Compound.* 1998;2:314–317.

Famotidine Suspension 8 mg/ml—Formulation 1

Ingredients:

Famotidine 40-mg tablet	24 tablets
Sterile Water for Irrigation	Small amount
Ora-Sweet/Ora-Plus*	**QSAD:** 120 ml

Preparation Details:

1. Triturate tablets to a fine powder in a mortar and pestle.
2. Levigate with Sterile Water for Irrigation to form a paste.
3. Add base solution in increasing amounts while mixing thoroughly.
4. Transfer contents of the mortar to a graduated cylinder.
5. Rinse the mortar and pestle with base solution and pour into graduated cylinder.
6. Add base solution to the graduated cylinder to achieve the total volume indicated above.
7. Transfer contents of the graduated cylinder into an appropriate size amber bottle.
8. Shake well to mix.

Storage Conditions: Room Temperature

Special Instructions: *Mix 60 ml of Ora-Sweet with 60 ml of Ora-Plus. Use mixture as base solution. Shake well before use.

Commercially Available: Use extemporaneously prepared formulation only when commercial product is unavailable.

Study Container Type: Plastic

Expiration Date: 95 days

References

1. Dentinger PJ, Swenson CF, Anaizi NH. Stability of famotidine in an extemporaneously compounded oral liquid. *Am J Health-Syst Pharm.* 2000;57:1340–1342.

Famotidine Syrup 8 mg/ml—Formulation 2

Ingredients:

Famotidine 40-mg tablet	24 tablets
Sterile Water for Irrigation	40 ml
Cherry Syrup	**QSAD:** 120 ml

Preparation Details:

1. Triturate tablets to a fine powder in a mortar and pestle.
2. Levigate with 20 ml of Sterile Water for Irrigation to form a paste.
3. Add base solution in increasing amounts while mixing thoroughly.
4. Transfer contents of the mortar to a graduated cylinder.
5. Rinse the mortar and pestle with 20 ml of Sterile Water for Irrigation and pour into graduated cylinder.
6. Add base solution to the graduated cylinder to achieve the total volume indicated above.
7. Transfer contents of the graduated cylinder into an appropriate size amber bottle.
8. Shake well to mix.

Storage Conditions: Refrigerate

Special Instructions: Expiration date of 15 days when stored at room temperature. Shake well before use.

Commercially Available: Use extemporaneously prepared formulation only when commercial product is unavailable.

Study Container Type: Glass

Expiration Date: 20 days

References

1. Quercia RA, Jay GT, Fan C, et al. Stability of famotidine in an extemporaneously prepared oral liquid. *Am J Hosp Pharm.* 1993;50:691–693.

Fluconazole Solution 1 mg/ml

Ingredients:

Fluconazole 100-mg tablet	1 tablet
Sterile Water for Irrigation	**QSAD:** 100 ml

Preparation Details:

1. Triturate tablet to a fine powder in a mortar and pestle.
2. Levigate with a small amount of base solution to form a paste.
3. Add base solution in increasing amounts while mixing thoroughly.
4. Transfer contents of the mortar to a graduated cylinder.
5. Rinse the mortar and pestle with base solution and pour into graduated cylinder.
6. Add base solution to the graduated cylinder to achieve the total volume indicated above.
7. Transfer contents of the graduated cylinder into an appropriate size amber bottle.
8. Shake well to mix.

Storage Conditions: Room Temperature or Refrigerate

Special Instructions: Shake well before use.

Commercially Available (as a 10-mg/ml and 40-mg/ml suspension): Use extemporaneously prepared formulation only when commercial product is unavailable or a more dilute solution is desired.

Study Container Type: Glass

Expiration Date: 15 days

References

1. Yamreudeewong W, Lopez-Anaya A, Rappaport H. Stability of fluconazole in an extemporaneously prepared oral liquid. *Am J Hosp Pharm.* 1993;50:2366–2367.

Fluoxetine Syrup 1 mg/ml

Ingredients:

Fluoxetine 4-mg/ml solution   30 ml

Simple Syrup NF   **QSAD:** 120 ml

Preparation Details:

1. Measure the volume of Fluoxetine solution with a graduated cylinder.
2. Add base solution to the graduated cylinder to achieve the total volume indicated above.
3. Transfer contents of the graduated cylinder into an appropriate size amber bottle.
4. Shake well to mix.

Storage Conditions: Room Temperature or Refrigerate

Special Instructions: Shake well before use.

Alternatives: May substitute base solution with Simple Syrup BP, Sterile Water for Irrigation, Aromatic Elixir USP, or grape-cranberry drink (Cran-Grape, Ocean Spray Cranberries, Inc., Lakeville, MA).

Commercially Available (as a 4-mg/ml solution): Use extemporaneously prepared formulation only when a more dilute syrup is desired.

Study Container Type: Glass

Expiration Date: 56 days

References

1. Peterson JA, Risley DS, Anderson PN, et al. Stability of fluoxetine hydrochloride in fluoxetine solution diluted with common pharmaceutical diluents. *Am J Hosp Pharm.* 1994;51:1342–1345.

Fluoxetine Syrup 2 mg/ml

Ingredients:

Fluoxetine 4-mg/ml solution   60 ml

Simple Syrup NF   **QSAD:** 120 ml

Preparation Details:

1. Measure the volume of Fluoxetine solution with a graduated cylinder.
2. Add base solution to the graduated cylinder to achieve the total volume indicated above.
3. Transfer contents of the graduated cylinder into an appropriate size amber bottle.
4. Shake well to mix.

Storage Conditions: Room Temperature or Refrigerate

Special Instructions: Shake well before use.

Alternatives: May substitute base solution with Simple Syrup BP, Sterile Water for Irrigation, Aromatic Elixir USP, or grape-cranberry drink (Cran-Grape, Ocean Spray Cranberries, Inc., Lakeville, MA).

Commercially Available (as a 4-mg/ml solution): Use extemporaneously prepared formulation only when a more dilute syrup is desired.

Study Container Type: Glass

Expiration Date: 56 days

References

1. Peterson JA, Risley DS, Anderson PN, et al. Stability of fluoxetine hydrochloride in fluoxetine solution diluted with common pharmaceutical diluents. *Am J Hosp Pharm.* 1994;51:1342–1345.

Gabapentin Suspension 100 mg/ml

Ingredients:

Gabapentin 400-mg capsule   30 capsules

Ora-Sweet/Ora-Plus*   **QSAD:** 120 ml

Preparation Details:

1. Open capsules and empty contents into a mortar.
2. Triturate contents to a fine powder.
3. Levigate with a small amount of base solution to form a paste.
4. Add base solution in increasing amounts while mixing thoroughly.
5. Transfer contents of the mortar to a graduated cylinder.
6. Rinse the mortar and pestle with base solution and pour into graduated cylinder.
7. Add base solution to the graduated cylinder to achieve the total volume indicated above.
8. Transfer contents of the graduated cylinder into an appropriate size amber bottle.
9. Shake well to mix.

Storage Conditions: Room Temperature or Refrigerate

Special Instructions: *Mix 60 ml of Ora-Sweet with 60 ml of Ora-Plus. Use mixture as base solution. Expiration date of 56 days when stored at room temperature. Shake well before use.

Alternatives: May substitute base solution with 60 ml of Methylcellulose 1% (see page 60 for preparation directions) mixed with 60 ml of Simple Syrup NF.

Commercially Available (as a 50-mg/ml solution): Use extemporaneously prepared formulation only when a more concentrated suspension is desired.

Study Container Type: Plastic

Expiration Date: 90 days

References

1. Nahata MC. Development of two stable oral suspensions for gabapentin. *Pediatr Neurol.* 1999;20:195–197.

Granisetron Hydrochloride Suspension 0.05 mg/ml

Ingredients:

Granisetron 1-mg tablet	6 tablets
Ora-Sweet/Ora-Plus*	**QSAD:** 120 ml

Preparation Details:

1. Triturate tablets to a fine powder in a mortar and pestle.
2. Levigate with a small amount of base solution to form a paste.
3. Add base solution in increasing amounts while mixing thoroughly.
4. Transfer contents of the mortar to a graduated cylinder.
5. Rinse the mortar and pestle with base solution and pour into graduated cylinder.
6. Add base solution to the graduated cylinder to achieve the total volume indicated above.
7. Transfer contents of the graduated cylinder into an appropriate size amber bottle.
8. Shake well to mix.

Storage Conditions: Room Temperature or Refrigerate

Special Instructions: *Mix 60 ml of Ora-Sweet with 60 ml of Ora-Plus. Use mixture as base solution. Shake well before use.

Alternatives: May substitute base solution with 60 ml of Methylcellulose 1% (see page 60 for preparation directions) mixed with 60 ml of Simple Syrup NF.

Commercially Available (as a 0.2-mg/ml solution): Use extemporaneously prepared formulation only when a more dilute suspension is desired.

Study Container Type: Plastic

Expiration Date: 90 days

References

1. Nahata MC, Morosco RS, Hipple TF. Stability of granisetron hydrochloride in two oral suspensions. *Am J Health-Syst Pharm.* 1998;55:2511–2513.

Granisetron Hydrochloride Syrup 0.2 mg/ml

Ingredients:

Granisetron 1-mg tablet	24 tablets
Sterile Water for Irrigation	60 ml
Cherry Syrup	**QSAD:** 120 ml

Preparation Details:

1. Triturate tablets to a fine powder in a mortar and pestle.
2. Levigate with Sterile Water for Irrigation to form a paste.
3. Add Sterile Water for Irrigation in increasing amounts while mixing thoroughly.
4. Transfer contents of the mortar to a graduated cylinder.
5. Rinse the mortar and pestle with base solution and pour into graduated cylinder.
6. Add base solution to the graduated cylinder to achieve the total volume indicated above.
7. Transfer contents of the graduated cylinder into an appropriate size amber bottle.
8. Shake well to mix.

Storage Conditions: Room Temperature or Refrigerate

Special Instructions: Shake well before use.

Commercially Available: Use extemporaneously prepared formulation only when commercial product is unavailable.

Study Container Type: Plastic

Expiration Date: 14 days

References

1. Quercia RA, Zhang J, Fan C, et al. Stability of granisetron hydrochloride in an extemporaneously prepared oral liquid. *Am J Health-Syst Pharm*. 1997;54:1404–1406.

Indomethacin Syrup 2 mg/ml

Ingredients:

Indomethacin 50-mg capsule	4 capsules
Alcohol 98%	10 ml
Methylparaben powder	5 mg
Propylparaben powder	2 mg
Simple Syrup NF	**QSAD:** 100 ml

Preparation Details:

1. Open capsules and empty contents into a mortar.
2. Add Methylparaben and Propylparaben powder in the mortar
3. Triturate contents to a fine powder.
4. Levigate with Alcohol to form a paste.
5. Add base solution in increasing amounts while mixing thoroughly.
6. Transfer contents of the mortar to a graduated cylinder.
7. Rinse the mortar and pestle with base solution and pour into graduated cylinder.
8. Add base solution to the graduated cylinder to achieve the total volume indicated above.
9. Transfer contents of the graduated cylinder into an appropriate size amber bottle.
10. Shake well to mix.

Storage Conditions: Room Temperature

Special Instructions: Shake well before use.

Commercially Available (as a 5-mg/ml suspension): Use extemporaneously prepared formulation only when a more dilute syrup is desired.

Study Container Type: Unknown

Expiration Date: 224 days

References

1. Gupta VD, Gibbs CW, Ghanekar AG. Stability of pediatric liquid dosage forms of ethacrynic acid, indomethacin, methyldopa hydrochloride, prednisone and spironolactone. *Am J Hosp Pharm*. 1978;35:1382–1385.

Itraconazole Suspension 20 mg/ml

Ingredients:

Itraconazole 100-mg capsule	20 capsules
Alcohol 98%	7.5 ml
Ora-Sweet/Ora-Plus*	**QSAD:** 100 ml

Preparation Details:

1. Open capsules and empty contents into a mortar.
2. Add Alcohol to beads and let it stand for 3–4 minutes to soften the beads.
3. Triturate beads to a fine powder.
4. Levigate with a small amount of base solution to form a paste.
5. Add base solution in increasing amounts while mixing thoroughly.
6. Transfer contents of the mortar to a graduated cylinder.
7. Rinse the mortar and pestle with base solution and pour into graduated cylinder.
8. Add base solution to the graduated cylinder to achieve the total volume indicated above.
9. Transfer contents of the graduated cylinder into an appropriate size amber bottle.
10. Shake well to mix.

Storage Conditions: Room Temperature or Refrigerate

Special Instructions: *Mix 50 ml of Ora-Sweet with 50 ml of Ora-Plus. Use mixture as base solution. Shake well before use.

Commercially Available (as a 10-mg/ml solution): Use extemporaneously prepared formulation only when commercial product is unavailable or a more concentrated suspension is desired. Extemporaneously prepared suspension may not achieve same bioavailability as commercially available formulation. Monitoring of serum itraconazole concentration may be warranted.

Study Container Type: Plastic

Expiration Date: 56 days

References

1. Abdel-Rahman SM, Nahata MC. Stability of itraconazole in an extemporaneous suspension. *J Ped Pharm Prac.* 1998;3:115–118.
2. Villarreal JD, Erush SC. Bioavailability of itraconazole from oral liquids in question. *Am J Health-Syst Pharm.* 1995;52:1707–1708.
3. Christensen KJ, Gubbins PO, Gurley BJ, et al. Relative bioavailability of itraconazole from an extemporaneously prepared suspension and from the marketed capsules. *Am J Health-Syst Pharm. 1998;*55:261–265.

Itraconazole Syrup 40 mg/ml

Ingredients:

Itraconazole 100-mg capsule	48 capsules
Alcohol 98%	8–10 ml
Simple Syrup NF	**QSAD:** 120 ml

Preparation Details:

1. Open capsules and empty contents into a mortar.
2. Add Alcohol to beads and let it stand for 3–4 minutes to soften the beads.
3. Triturate beads to a fine powder.
4. Levigate with a small amount of base solution to form a paste.
5. Add base solution in increasing amounts while mixing thoroughly.
6. Transfer contents of the mortar to a graduated cylinder.
7. Rinse the mortar and pestle with base solution and pour into graduated cylinder.
8. Add base solution to the graduated cylinder to achieve the total volume indicated above.
9. Transfer contents of graduated cylinder into appropriate size amber bottle.
10. Shake well to mix.

Storage Conditions: Refrigerate

Special Instructions: Shake well before use.

Commercially Available (as a 10-mg/ml solution): Use extemporaneously prepared formulation only when commercial product is unavailable or a more concentrated syrup is desired. Extemporaneously prepared suspension may not achieve same bioavailability as commercially available formulation. Monitoring of serum itraconazole concentration may be warranted.

Study Container Type: Glass

Expiration Date: 35 days

References

1. Jacobson PA, Johnson CE, Walters JR. Stability of itraconazole in an extemporaneously compounded oral liquid. *J Health-Syst Pharm.* 1995;52:189–191.
2. Villarreal JD, Erush SC. Bioavailability of itraconazole from oral liquids in question. *Am J Health-Syst Pharm.* 1995;52:1701–1708.
3. Christensen KJ, Gubbins PO, Gurley BJ, et al. Relative bioavailability of itraconazole from an extemporaneously prepared suspension and from the marketed capsules. *Am J Health-Syst Pharm.* 1998;55:261–265.

Levofloxacin Suspension 50 mg/ml

Ingredients:

Levofloxacin 500-mg tablet	12 tablets
Strawberry Syrup NF/Ora-Plus*	**QSAD:** 120 ml

Preparation Details:

1. Triturate tablets to a fine powder in a mortar and pestle.
2. Levigate with a small amount of base solution to form a paste.
3. Add base solution in increasing amounts while mixing thoroughly.
4. Transfer contents of the mortar to a graduated cylinder.
5. Rinse the mortar and pestle with base solution and pour into graduated cylinder.
6. Add base solution to the graduated cylinder to achieve the total volume indicated above.
7. Transfer contents of the graduated cylinder into an appropriate size amber bottle.
8. Shake well to mix.

Storage Conditions: Room Temperature or Refrigerate

Special Instructions: *Mix 60 ml of Strawberry Syrup NF with 60 ml of Ora-Plus. Use mixture as base solution. Shake well before use.

Commercially Available (as a 25-mg/ml solution): Use extemporaneously prepared formulation only when commercial product is unavailable or a more concentrated suspension is desired.

Study Container Type: Plastic

Expiration Date: 57 days

References

1. VandenBussche HL, Johnson CE, Fontana EM, et al. Stability of levofloxacin in an extemporaneously compounded oral liquid. *Am J Health-Syst Pharm.* 1999;56:2316–2318.

Midazolam Gelatin 1 mg/ml

Ingredients:

Midazolam 5-mg/ml injection	45 ml
Purified Water, USP	**QSAD:** 225 ml

Preparation Details:

1. Measure 180 ml of water and add to beaker. Heat to boiling.
2. Add 3 oz of flavored gelatin to water and stir until dissolved.
3. Allow solution to cool to room temperature. Initial pH of gelatin solution should be approximately 4.
4. Add injectable solution and stir well.
5. Accurately measure desired volume of solution and place in unit-dose plastic cups.
6. Place cups in refrigerator and allow gelatin to become firm (1–2 hours).

Storage Conditions: Refrigerate

Special Instructions: Label appropriately and place in a food storage bag in refrigerator. Expiration date of 28 days when stored at –20°C.

Commercially Available (as a 2-mg/ml syrup): Use extemporaneously prepared formulation only when a more dilute concentration is desired.

Study Container Type: Plastic

Expiration Date: 14 days

References

1. Bhatt-Mehta V, Johnson CE, Kostoff L, et al. Stability of midazolam hydrochloride in extemporaneously prepared flavored gelatin. *Am J Hosp Pharm.* 1993;50:472–475.

Midazolam Gelatin 2 mg/ml

Ingredients:

Midazolam 5-mg/ml injection	90 ml
Purified Water, USP	**QSAD:** 225 ml

Preparation Details:

1. Measure 135 ml of water and add to beaker. Heat to boiling.
2. Add 3 oz of flavored gelatin to water and stir until dissolved.
3. Allow solution to cool to room temperature. Initial pH of gelatin solution should be approximately 4.
4. Add injectable solution and stir well.
5. Accurately measure desired volume of solution and place in unit dose plastic cups.
6. Place cups in refrigerator and allow gelatin to become firm (1–2 hours).

Storage Conditions: Refrigerate

Special Instructions: Label appropriately and place in a food storage bag in refrigerator. Expiration date of 28 days when stored at –20°C.

Commercially Available (as a 2-mg/ml syrup): Use extemporaneously prepared formulation only when commercial product is unavailable or a more dilute concentration is desired.

Study Container Type: Plastic

Expiration Date: 14 days

References

1. Bhatt-Mehta V, Johnson CE, Kostoff L, et al. Stability of midazolam hydrochloride in extemporaneously prepared flavored gelatin. *Am J Hosp Pharm.* 1993;50:472–475.

Midazolam Syrup 2.5 mg/ml

Ingredients:

Midazolam 5-mg/ml injection   60 ml

Syrpalta, dye-free   **QSAD:** 120 ml

Preparation Details:

1. Withdraw volume of injectable solution using a 60-ml syringe.
2. Transfer the solution to a graduated cylinder.
3. Add base solution to the graduated cylinder to achieve the total volume indicated above.
4. Transfer contents of the graduated cylinder into an appropriate size amber bottle.
5. Shake well to mix.

Storage Conditions: Room Temperature or Refrigerate

Special Instructions: Shake well before use.

Commercially Available (as a 2-mg/ml syrup): Use extemporaneously prepared formulation only when commercial product is unavailable or a more concentrated syrup is desired.

Study Container Type: Glass

Expiration Date: 56 days

References

1. Steedman SL, Koonce JR, Wynn JE, et al. Stability of midazolam hydrochloride in a flavored, dye-free oral solution. *Am J Hosp Pharm.* 1992;49:615–618.

Mycophenolate Mofetil Suspension 50 mg/ml

Ingredients:

Mycophenolate Mofetil 250-mg capsule	24 capsules
Ora-Plus	30 ml
Cherry Syrup	**QSAD:** 120 ml

Preparation Details:

Must be prepared in a vertical hood. Must wear mask during preparation.

1. Open capsules and empty contents into a mortar.
2. Triturate contents to a fine powder.
3. Levigate with 30 ml of Ora-Plus to form paste.
4. Add base solution in increasing amounts while mixing thoroughly.
5. Transfer contents of the mortar to a graduated cylinder.
6. Rinse the mortar and pestle with base solution and pour into graduated cylinder.
7. Add base solution to the graduated cylinder to achieve the total volume indicated above.
8. Transfer contents of graduated cylinder into appropriate size amber bottle.
9. Shake well to mix.

Storage Conditions: Refrigerate

Special Instructions: Shake well before use. Caution teratogenic agent.

Commercially Available (as a 200-mg/ml suspension): Use extemporaneously prepared formulation only when commercial product is unavailable or a more dilute suspension is desired.

Study Container Type: Unknown

Expiration Date: 210 days

References

1. Venkataramanan R, McCombs J, Zuckerman S, et al. Stability of mycophenolate mofetil as an extemporaneous suspension. *Ann Pharmacother.* 1998;32:755–757.

Mycophenolate Mofetil Syrup 100 mg/ml

Ingredients:

Mycophenolate Mofetil 250-mg capsule	48 capsules
Sterile Water for Irrigation	Small amount
Cherry Syrup	**QSAD:** 120 ml

Preparation Details:

Must be prepared in a vertical hood. Must wear mask during preparation.

1. Open capsules and empty contents into a mortar.
2. Triturate contents to a fine powder.
3. Levigate with Sterile Water for Irrigation to form a paste.
4. Add base solution in increasing amounts while mixing thoroughly.
5. Transfer contents of the mortar to a graduated cylinder.
6. Rinse the mortar and pestle with base solution and pour into graduated cylinder.
7. Add base solution to the graduated cylinder to achieve the total volume indicated above.
8. Transfer contents of graduated cylinder into appropriate size amber bottle.
9. Shake well to mix.

Storage Conditions: Room Temperature or Refrigerate

Special Instructions: Shake well before use. Caution teratogenic agent.

Alternatives: May substitute base solution with Ora-Plus 120 ml with artificial cherry flavoring 0.48 ml, 10% FD&C Red No. 40 0.06 ml, aspartame 360 mg with an expiration date of 28 days when stored at room temperature.

Commercially Available (as a 200-mg/ml suspension): Use extemporaneously prepared formulation only when commercial product is unavailable or a more dilute syrup is desired.

Study Container Type: Plastic

Expiration Date: 120 days

References

1. Anaizi NH, Swenson CF, Dentinger PJ. Stability of mycophenolate mofetil in an extemporaneously compounded oral liquid. *Am J Health-Syst Pharm.* 1998;55:926–929.
2. Swenson CF, Dentinger PJ, Anaizi NH. Stability of mycophenolate mofetil in an extemporaneously compounded sugar-free oral liquid. *Am J Health-Syst Pharm.* 1999;56: 2224–2226.

Nizatidine Solution 2.5 mg/ml

Ingredients:

Nizatidine 300-mg capsule   1 capsule

Sterile Water for Irrigation   **QSAD:** 120 ml

Preparation Details:

1. Open capsule and empty contents into a mortar.
2. Triturate contents to a fine powder.
3. Levigate with a small amount of base solution to form a paste.
4. Add base solution in increasing amounts while mixing thoroughly.
5. Transfer contents of the mortar to a graduated cylinder.
6. Rinse the mortar and pestle with base solution and pour into graduated cylinder.
7. Add base solution to the graduated cylinder to achieve the total volume indicated above.
8. Transfer contents of graduated cylinder into appropriate size amber bottle.
9. Shake well to mix.

Storage Conditions: Room Temperature or Refrigerate

Special Instructions: Shake well before use.

Alternatives: May substitute base solution with Gatorade Thirst Quencher Lemon Lime, Ocean Spray Cran-Grape Grape Cranberry Drink, Speas Farm Apple Juice, V8 100% Vegetable Juice, or Maalox.

Commercially Available (as a 15-mg/ml solution): Use extemporaneously prepared formulation only when commercial product is unavailable or a more dilute solution is desired. Expiration date for all alternative base solutions is 2 days room temperature or refrigerate except for Ocean Spray Cran-Grape Grape Cranberry Drink (8 hours room temperature, 2 days refrigerate) and V8 100% Vegetable Juice (1 day room temperature, 2 days refrigerate).

Study Container Type: Unknown

Expiration Date: 2 days

References

1. Lantz MD, Wozniak TJ. Stability of nizatidine in extemporaneous oral liquid preparations. *Am J Hosp Pharm.* 1990;47:2716–2719.

Ondansetron Suspension 0.8 mg/ml

Ingredients:

Ondansetron 8-mg tablet	12 tablets
Ora-Plus	60 ml
Ora-Sweet	**QSAD:** 120 ml

Preparation Details:

1. Triturate tablets to a fine powder in a mortar and pestle.
2. Levigate with a small amount of Ora-Plus to form paste.
3. Add base solution in increasing amounts while mixing thoroughly.
4. Transfer contents of the mortar to a graduated cylinder.
5. Rinse the mortar and pestle with base solution and pour into graduated cylinder.
6. Add base solution to the graduated cylinder to achieve the total volume indicated above.
7. Transfer contents of the graduated cylinder into an appropriate size amber bottle.
8. Shake well to mix.

Storage Conditions: Refrigerate

Special Instructions: Shake well before use.

Alternatives: May substitute base solution with cherry syrup, Syrpalta, or Ora-Sweet SF.

Commercially Available: Use extemporaneously prepared formulation only when commercial product is unavailable.

Study Container Type: Plastic

Expiration Date: 42 days

References

1. Williams CL, Sanders PL, Laizure SC, et al. Stability of ondansetron hydrochloride in syrups compounded from tablets. *Am J Hosp Pharm.* 1994;51:806–809.

Oseltamivir Syrup 15 mg/ml

Ingredients:

Oseltamivir 75-mg capsule   12 capsules

Ora-Sweet SF   **QSAD:** 60 ml

Preparation Details:

1. Open capsules and empty contents into a mortar.
2. Triturate contents to a fine powder.
3. Levigate with a small amount of base solution to form a paste.
4. Add base solution in increasing amounts while mixing thoroughly.
5. Transfer contents of the mortar to a graduated cylinder.
6. Rinse the mortar and pestle with base solution and pour into graduated cylinder.
7. Add base solution to the graduated cylinder to achieve the total volume indicated above.
8. Transfer contents of graduated cylinder into appropriate size amber bottle.
9. Shake well to mix.

Storage Conditions: Refrigerate

Special Instructions: Expiration date of 5 days when stored at room temperature. Shake well before use.

Alternatives: May substitute base solution with cherry syrup.

Commercially Available (as a 12-mg/ml suspension): Use extemporaneously prepared formulation only when commercial product is unavailable or a more concentrated syrup is desired.

Study Container Type: Glass and plastic

Expiration Date: 35 days

References

1. Winiarski AP, Infeld MH, Tscherne R, et al. Preparation and stability of extemporaneous oral liquid formulations of oseltamivir using commercially available capsules. *J Am Pharm Assoc.* 2007;47:747–755.

Phenobarbital Suspension 10 mg/ml

Ingredients:

Phenobarbital 60-mg tablet   20 tablets

Ora-Sweet/Ora-Plus*   **QSAD:** 120 ml

Preparation Details:

1. Triturate tablets to a fine powder in a mortar and pestle.
2. Levigate with a small amount of base solution to form a paste.
3. Add base solution in increasing amounts while mixing thoroughly.
4. Transfer contents of the mortar to a graduated cylinder.
5. Rinse the mortar and pestle with base solution and pour into graduated cylinder.
6. Add base solution to the graduated cylinder to achieve the total volume indicated above.
7. Transfer contents of graduated cylinder into appropriate size amber bottle.
8. Shake well to mix.

Storage Conditions: Room Temperature

Special Instructions: *Mix 60 ml of Ora-Plus with 60 ml of Ora-Sweet. Use mixture as base solution. Shake well before use.

Alternatives: May substitute base solution with 60 ml of Ora-Plus mixed with 60 ml of Ora-Sweet SF.

Commercially Available (as a 4-mg/ml elixir): Use extemporaneously prepared formulation only when commercial product is unavailable or a more concentrated alcohol-free suspension is desired. Bitter aftertaste. May administer chocolate syrup before medication administration or mix the preparation with chocolate syrup (1:1 by volume) immediately before administration to mask the bitter aftertaste.

Study Container Type: Plastic

Expiration Date: 115 days

References

1. Cober MP, Johnson CE. Stability of an extemporaneously prepared alcohol-free phenobarbital suspension. *Am J Health-Syst Pharm.* 2007;64:644–646.

Prednisolone Disodium Phosphate Solution 10 mg/ml

Ingredients:

Prednisolone Disodium Phosphate powder	1000 mg
Methylparaben powder	65 mg
Propylparaben powder	35 mg
Orange Syrup	40 ml
Sterile Water for Irrigation	**QSAD:** 100 ml

Preparation Details:

1. Weigh out Prednisolone Disodium Phosphate powder and place in mortar.
2. Triturate contents to a fine powder.
3. Add Methylparaben and Propylparaben powder in the mortar
4. Levigate with Orange Syrup to form paste.
5. Add base solution in increasing amounts while mixing thoroughly.
6. Transfer contents of the mortar to a graduated cylinder.
7. Rinse the mortar and pestle with base solution and pour into graduated cylinder.
8. Add base solution to the graduated cylinder to achieve the total volume indicated above.
9. Transfer contents of graduated cylinder into appropriate size amber bottle.
10. Shake well to mix.

Storage Conditions: Room Temperature

Special Instructions: Shake well before use.

Commercially Available (as a 1-mg/ml solution, 2-mg/ml solution, 3-mg/ml solution, and 4-mg/ml solution): Use extemporaneously prepared formulation only when commercial product is unavailable or a more concentrated solution is desired.

Study Container Type: Glass

Expiration Date: 270 days

References

1. Sullivan JA, Hobson LT. Prednisolone disodium phosphate stability in a prednisolone oral solution. *Aust J Hosp Pharm.* 1994;24:397–398.

Prednisone Syrup 0.5 mg/ml

Ingredients:

Prednisone 10-mg tablet	5 tablets
Sodium Benzoate	100 mg
Alcohol 98%	10 ml
Simple Syrup	**QSAD:** 100 ml

Preparation Details:

1. Triturate tablets to a fine powder in a mortar and pestle.
2. Add Sodium Benzoate powder in the mortar.
3. Levigate with Alcohol to form a paste.
4. Add base solution in increasing amounts while mixing thoroughly.
5. Transfer contents of the mortar to a graduated cylinder.
6. Rinse the mortar and pestle with base solution and pour into graduated cylinder.
7. Add base solution to the graduated cylinder to achieve the total volume indicated above.
8. Transfer contents of graduated cylinder into appropriate size amber bottle.
9. Shake well to mix.

Storage Conditions: Room Temperature

Special Instructions: Shake well before use.

Commercially Available (as a 1-mg/ml solution and 5-mg/ml solution): Use extemporaneously prepared formulation only when commercial product is unavailable or a more dilute syrup is desired.

Study Container Type: Unknown

Expiration Date: 84 days

References

1. Gupta VD, Gibbs CW, Ghanekar AG. Stability of pediatric liquid dosage forms of ethacrynic acid, indomethacin, methyldopate hydrochloride, prednisone and spironolactone. *Am J Hosp Pharm.* 1978;35:1382–1385.

Propranolol Syrup 1 mg/ml

Ingredients:

Propranolol 40-mg tablet   3 tablets

Simple Syrup   **QSAD:** 120 ml

Preparation Details:

1. Triturate tablets to a fine powder in a mortar and pestle.
2. Levigate with a small amount of base solution to form a paste.
3. Add base solution in increasing amounts while mixing thoroughly.
4. Transfer contents of the mortar to a graduated cylinder.
5. Rinse the mortar and pestle with base solution and pour into graduated cylinder.
6. Add base solution to the graduated cylinder to achieve the total volume indicated above.
7. Transfer contents of graduated cylinder into appropriate size amber bottle.
8. Shake well to mix.

Storage Conditions: Room Temperature

Special Instructions: Shake well before use.

Commercially Available (as a 4-mg/ml solution and 8-mg/ml solution): Use extemporaneously prepared formulation only when commercial product is unavailable or a more dilute syrup is desired.

Study Container Type: Glass

Expiration Date: 238 days

References

1. Gupta VD, Stewart KR. Stability of propranolol hydrochloride suspension and solution compounded from injection or tablets. *Am J Hosp Pharm.* 1987;44:360–361.

Ranitidine Syrup 15 mg/ml

Ingredients:

Ranitidine 150-mg tablet	12 tablets
Water (Distilled)/Simple Syrup*	**QSAD:** 120 ml

Preparation Details:

1. Triturate tablets to a fine powder in a mortar and pestle.
2. Levigate with a small amount of base solution to form a paste.
3. Add base solution in increasing amounts while mixing thoroughly.
4. Transfer contents of the mortar to a graduated cylinder.
5. Rinse the mortar and pestle with base solution and pour into graduated cylinder.
6. Add base solution to the graduated cylinder to achieve the total volume indicated above.
7. Transfer contents of the graduated cylinder into an appropriate size amber bottle.
8. Shake well to mix.

Storage Conditions: Room Temperature

Special Instructions: *Mix 60 ml of Water (Distilled) with 60 ml of Simple Syrup. Use mixture as base solution. Shake well before use.

Commercially Available: Use extemporaneously prepared formulation only when commercial product is unavailable.

Study Container Type: Unknown

Expiration Date: 7 days

References

1. Karnes HT, Harris SR, Garnett WR, et al. Concentration uniformity of extemporaneously prepared ranitidine suspension. *Am J Health-Syst Pharm.* 1989;46:304–307.

Tacrolimus Cream 0.1%

Ingredients:

Tacrolimus 5-mg capsule	12 capsules
Eucerin cream	**QSAD:** 60 g

Preparation Details:

1. Open capsules and empty contents on a glass plate.
2. Weigh out 60 g of Eucerin cream and place on the glass plate.
3. Levigate the powder into the Eucerin cream to make a homogenous cream.
4. Transfer contents on the glass plate into a 60-g ointment jar.

Storage Conditions: Room Temperature

Special Instructions: For external use only.

Commercially Available: Use extemporaneously prepared formulation only when commercial product is unavailable.

Study Container Type: Unknown

Expiration Date: 30 days

References

1. Verbal communications from Fujisawa, 1999.

Theophylline Suspension 5 mg/ml

Ingredients:

Theophylline 300-mg extend release tablet 2 tablets

Ora-Sweet/Ora-Plus*   **QSAD:** 120 ml

Preparation Details:

1. Triturate tablets to a fine powder in a mortar and pestle.
2. Levigate with a small amount of base solution to form a paste.
3. Add base solution in increasing amounts while mixing thoroughly.
4. Transfer contents of the mortar to a graduated cylinder.
5. Rinse the mortar and pestle with base solution and pour into graduated cylinder.
6. Add base solution to the graduated cylinder to achieve the total volume indicated above.
7. Transfer contents of the graduated cylinder into an appropriate size amber bottle.
8. Shake well to mix.

Storage Conditions: Room Temperature

Special Instructions: *Mix 60 ml of Ora-Plus with 60 ml of Ora-Sweet. Use mixture as base solution. Shake well before use.

Alternatives: May substitute base solution with 60 ml of Ora-Sweet SF mixed with 60 ml of Ora-Plus.

Commercially Available (as a 5.3-mg/ml elixir): Use extemporaneously prepared formulation only when commercial product is unavailable or a more dilute, alcohol-free suspension is desired.

Study Container Type: Plastic

Expiration Date: 90 days

References

1. Johnson CE, VanDeKoppel S, Myers E. Stability of anhydrous theophylline in extemporaneously prepared alcohol-free oral suspensions. *Am J Health-Syst Pharm.* 2005;62:2518–2520.

Trimethoprim Syrup 10 mg/ml

Ingredients:

Trimethoprim 100-mg tablet   12 tablets

Simple Syrup   **QSAD:** 120 ml

Preparation Details:

1. Triturate tablets to a fine powder in a mortar and pestle.
2. Levigate with a small amount of base solution to form a paste.
3. Add base solution in increasing amounts while mixing thoroughly.
4. Transfer contents of the mortar to a graduated cylinder.
5. Rinse the mortar and pestle with base solution and pour into graduated cylinder.
6. Add base solution to the graduated cylinder to achieve the total volume indicated above.
7. Transfer contents of the graduated cylinder into an appropriate size amber bottle.
8. Shake well to mix.

Storage Conditions: Refrigerate

Special Instructions: Shake well before use.

Commercially Available: Use extemporaneously prepared formulation only when commercial product is unavailable.

Study Container Type: Unknown

Expiration Date: 90 days

References

1. Nahata MC, Morosco RS, Hipple TF. Stability of trimethoprim in an extemporaneously prepared suspension. *J Pediatric Pharm Pract.* 1997;2:82–84.

Valganciclovir Suspension 30 mg/ml

Ingredients:

Valganciclovir 450-mg tablet   8 tablets

Ora-Sweet/Ora-Plus*   **QSAD:** 120 ml

Preparation Details:

Must be prepared in a vertical hood. Must wear mask during preparation.

1. Triturate tablets to a fine powder in a mortar and pestle.
2. Levigate with a small amount of base solution to form a paste.
3. Add base solution in increasing amounts while mixing thoroughly.
4. Transfer contents of the mortar to a graduated cylinder.
5. Rinse the mortar and pestle with base solution and pour into graduated cylinder.
6. Add base solution to the graduated cylinder to achieve the total volume indicated above.
7. Transfer contents of graduated cylinder into appropriate size amber bottle.
8. Shake well to mix.

Storage Conditions: Refrigerate

Special Instructions: *Mix 60 ml of Ora-Sweet with 60 ml of Ora-Plus. Use mixture as base solution. Shake well before use.

Commercially Available (as a 50-mg/ml suspension): Use extemporaneously prepared formulation only when commercial product is unavailable or a more dilute suspension is desired.

Study Container Type: Glass

Expiration Date: 35 days

References

1. Henkin CC, Griener JC, Ten Eick AP. Stability of valganciclovir in extemporaneously compounded liquid formulations. *Am J Health-Syst Pharm.* 2003;60:687–690.

Valganciclovir Suspension 60 mg/ml

Ingredients:

Valganciclovir 450-mg tablet   16 tablets

Ora-Sweet/Ora-Plus*   **QSAD:** 120 ml

Preparation Details:

Must be prepared in a vertical hood. Must wear mask during preparation.

1. Triturate tablets to a fine powder in a mortar and pestle.
2. Levigate with a small amount of base solution to form a paste.
3. Add base solution in increasing amounts while mixing thoroughly.
4. Transfer contents of the mortar to a graduated cylinder.
5. Rinse the mortar and pestle with base solution and pour into graduated cylinder.
6. Add base solution to the graduated cylinder to achieve the total volume indicated above.
7. Transfer contents of the graduated cylinder into an appropriate size amber bottle.
8. Shake well to mix.

Storage Conditions: Refrigerate

Special Instructions: *Mix 60 ml of Ora-Sweet with 60 ml of Ora-Plus. Use mixture as base solution. Shake well before use.

Commercially Available (as a 50-mg/ml suspension): Use extemporaneously prepared formulation only when commercial product is unavailable or a more concentrated suspension is desired.

Study Container Type: Glass

Expiration Date: 35 days

References

1. Henkin CC, Griener JC, Ten Eick AP. Stability of valganciclovir in extemporaneously compounded liquid formulations. *Am J Health-Syst Pharm.* 2003;60:687–690.

Zidovudine Syrup 10 mg/ml

Ingredients:

Zidovudine 100-mg capsule	12 capsules
Simple Syrup	**QSAD:** 120 ml

Preparation Details:

1. Open capsules and empty contents into a mortar.
2. Triturate contents to a fine powder.
3. Levigate with a small amount of base solution to form a paste.
4. Add base solution in increasing amounts while mixing thoroughly.
5. Transfer contents of the mortar to a graduated cylinder.
6. Rinse the mortar and pestle with base solution and pour into graduated cylinder.
7. Add base solution to the graduated cylinder to achieve the total volume indicated above.
8. Transfer contents of the graduated cylinder into an appropriate size amber bottle.
9. Shake well to mix.

Storage Conditions: Room Temperature

Special Instructions: Shake well before use.

Commercially Available: Use extemporaneously prepared formulation only when commercial product is unavailable.

Study Container Type: Glass

Expiration Date: 90 days

References

1. Radwan MA. Stability indicating HPLC assay of zidovudine in extemporaneous syrup. *Analytical Letter.* 1994;27:1159–1164.

Appendices

ASHP Technical Assistance Bulletin on Compounding Nonsterile Products in Pharmacies

Introduction

Pharmacists are the only health care providers formally trained in the art and science of compounding medications.[1,2] Therefore pharmacists are expected, by the medical community and the public, to possess the knowledge and skills necessary to compound extemporaneous preparations. Pharmacists have a responsibility to provide compounding services for patients with unique drug product needs.

This Technical Assistance Bulletin is intended to assist pharmacists in the extemporaneous compounding of nonsterile drug products for individual patients. Included in this document is information on facilities and equipment, ingredient selection, training, documentation and record keeping, stability and beyond-use dating, packaging and labeling, and limited batch compounding. This document is not intended for manufacturers or licensed repackagers.

Facilities and Equipment

Facilities. It is not necessary that compounding activities be located in a separate facility; however, the compounding area should be located sufficiently away from routine dispensing and counseling functions and high traffic areas. The area should be isolated from potential interruptions, chemical contaminants, and sources of dust and particulate matter. To minimize chemical contaminants, the immediate area and work counter should be free of previously used drugs and chemicals. To minimize dust and particulate matter, cartons and boxes should not be stored or opened in the compounding area. The compounding area should not contain dust-collecting overhangs (e.g., ceiling utility pipes, hanging light fixtures) and ledges (e.g., windowsills). Additionally, at least one sink should be located in or near the compounding area for hand washing before compounding operations. Proper temperature and humidity control within the compounding area or facility is desirable.

Work areas should be well lighted, and work surfaces should be level and clean. The work surface should be smooth, impervious, free of cracks and crevices (preferably seamless), and nonshedding. Surfaces should be cleaned at both the beginning and the end of each distinct compounding operation with an appropriate cleaner or solvent. The entire compounding facility should be cleaned daily or weekly (as needed) but not during the actual process of compounding.

Equipment. The equipment needed to compound a drug product depends upon the particular dosage form requested. Although boards of pharmacy publish lists of required equipment and accessories, these lists are not intended to limit the equipment available to pharmacists for compounding.[2] Equipment should be maintained in good working order. Pharmacists are responsible for obtaining the required equipment and accessories and ensuring that equipment is properly maintained and maintenance is documented.

Weighing Equipment. In addition to a torsion balance, pharmacists who routinely compound may need to use a top-loading electronic balance that has a capacity of at least 300 g, a sensitivity of ±1 mg (or 0.1 mg), and 1-mg, 100-mg, 1-g, and 100-g weights for checking. Balances should be maintained in areas of low humidity and should be stored on flat, nonvibrating surfaces away from drafts. At least annually, the performance of balances should be checked according to the guidelines found in *Remington's Pharmaceutical Sciences,*[3] *USP XXII NF XVII: The United States Pharmacopeia–The National Formulary (USP–NF),*[4] or *USP DI Volume III: Approved Drug Products and Legal Requirements*[5] or the instructions of the balance manufacturer. Performance should be documented.

Weights should be stored in rigid, compartmentalized boxes and handled with metal, plastic, or plastic-tipped forceps—not fingers—to avoid scratching or soiling. Since most Class III prescription balances are only accurate to ±5 or 10 mg, Class P weights may be used for compounding purposes.[4] The *USP–NF* recommends that the class of weights used be chosen to limit the error to 0.1%. In practical terms this means that Class P weights can be used for weighing quantities greater than 100 mg.

The minimum weighable quantity must be determined for any balance being used for compounding. To avoid errors of 5% or more on a Class III balance with a sensitivity requirement of 6 mg, quantities of less than 120 mg of any substance should not be weighed. Smaller quantities may be weighed on more sensitive balances. If an amount is needed that is less than the minimum weighable quantity determined for a balance, an aliquot method of measurement should be used.

Measuring Equipment. The pharmacist should use judgment in selecting measuring equipment. The recommendations given in the *USP–NF* General Information section on volumetric apparatus should be followed. For maximum accuracy in measuring liquids, a pharmacist should select a graduate with a capacity equal to or slightly larger than the volume to be measured. The general rule is to measure no less than 20% of the capacity of a graduate. Calibrated syringes of the appropriate size may be preferred over graduated cylinders for measuring viscous liquids such as glycerin or mineral oil, since these liquids drain slowly and incompletely from graduated cylinders. Viscous liquids may also be weighed if this is more convenient, provided that the appropriate conversions from volume to weight are made by using the specific gravity of the liquid. Thick, opaque liquids should be weighed. For example, if a formulation specifies 1.5 mL of a liquid, it is better to use a 3-mL syringe with appropriate graduations to measure 1.5 mL than to use a 10-mL graduated cylinder, since quantities of less than 2.0 mL cannot be accurately measured in a 10-mL graduate. Also, if an opaque, viscous chemical, such as Coal Tar, USP, must be measured, it is more accurate to weigh the substance than to try to read a meniscus on a graduated cylinder or a fill line on a syringe.

For volumes smaller than 1 mL, micropipettes are recommended, in sizes to cover the range of volumes measured. Two or three variable pipettes can usually cover the range from about 50 µL to 1 mL.

Although conical graduates are convenient for mixing solutions, the error in reading the bottom of the meniscus increases as the sides flare toward the top of the graduate. Therefore, for accurate measurements, cylindrical graduates are preferred. Conical graduates having a capacity of less than 25 mL should not be used in prescription compounding.[4]

Compounding Equipment. Pharmacists need at least two types of mortars and pestles—one glass and one Wedgwood or porcelain. The sizes of each will depend on the drug products being compounded. Glass mortars should be used for liquid preparations (solutions and suspensions) and for mixing chemicals that stain or are oily. Generally, glass mortars should be used for

antineoplastic agents. Because of their rough surface, Wedgwood mortars are preferred for reducing the size of dry crystals and hard powder particles and for preparing emulsions. Porcelain mortars have a smoother surface than Wedgwood mortars and are ideal for blending powders and pulverizing soft aggregates or crystals. When Wedgwood mortars are used for small amounts of crystals or powders, the inside surface may first be lightly dusted with lactose to fill any crevices in which the crystals or powders might lodge. If the contact surfaces of the mortar and pestle become smooth with use, rubbing them with a small amount of sand or emery powder may adequately roughen them. Over extended use, a pestle and a mortar become shaped to each other's curvature. Thus, to ensure maximum contact between the surface of the head of each pestle and the interior of its corresponding mortar, pestles and mortars should not be interchanged.[3]

The compounding area should be stocked with appropriate supplies. Although supply selection depends on the types of products compounded, all areas should have weighing papers, weighing cups, or both to protect balance pans and spatulas. Glassine weighing papers (as opposed to bond weighing paper) should be used for products such as ointments, creams, and some dry chemicals. Disposable weighing dishes should also be stocked for substances like Coal Tar, USP.

Each compounding area should have stainless steel and plastic spatulas for mixing ointments and creams and handling dry chemicals. The pharmacist should exercise judgment in selecting the size and type of spatula. Small spatula blades (6 inches long or less) are preferred for handling dry chemicals, but larger spatula blades (>6 inches) are preferred for large amounts of ointments or creams and for preparing compactible powder blends for capsules. Plastic spatulas should be used for chemicals that may react with stainless steel blades. A variety of spatulas should be stocked in the compounding area, including 4-, 6-, and 8-inch stainless steel spatulas (one each) and 4- and 6-inch plastic spatulas (one each). Imprinted spatulas should not be used in compounding, since the imprinted ink on the spatula blade may contaminate the product.

The compounding area should contain an ointment slab, pill tile, or parchment ointment pad. Although parchment ointment pads are convenient and reduce cleanup time, parchment paper cannot be used for the preparation of creams because it will absorb water. Therefore, an ointment slab or pill tile is necessary. If supposi-tories are compounded, appropriate suppository molds, either reusable or disposable, should be available.

Other useful equipment and supplies may include funnels, filter paper, beakers, glass stirring rods, a source of heat (hot plate or microwave oven), a refrigerator, and a freezer—in some cases, an ultrafreezer capable of maintain-ing temperatures as low as −80 °C.

Ingredients

Ideally, only USP or NF chemicals manufactured by FDA-inspected manufacturers should be used for compounding. Although chemicals labeled USP or NF meet *USP–NF* standards for strength, quality, and purity for human drug products, the facilities in which the chemicals were manufac-tured may not meet FDA Good Manufacturing Practice (GMP) standards. In the event that a needed chemical is not available from an FDA-inspected facility, the pharmacist should, by next best preference, obtain a USP or NF product. If that is not available, the pharmacist should use professional judgment and may have to obtain the highest-grade chemical possible. Chemical grades that may be considered in this situation are ACS grade (meeting or exceeding specifica-tions listed for reagent chemicals by the American Chemical Society) and FCC grade (meeting or exceeding requirements defined by the Food Chemicals Codex). Additional professional judgment is especially necessary in cases of chemical substances that have not been approved for *any* medical use. Particularly in these cases, but also in others as needed, the pharmacist, prescriber, and patient should be well informed of the risks involved.

Selection of ingredients may also depend on the dosage form to be compounded. In most cases, the prescriber specifies a particular dosage form, such as a topical ointment, oral solution or rectal suppository. Sometimes, however, the prescriber relies on the pharmacist to decide on an appropriate form. Irrespective of how the drug order is written, the pharmacist should evaluate the appropriateness of ingredients and the drug delivery system recommended. Factors to consider in selecting the dosage form include (1) physical and chemical characteristics of the active ingredient, (2) possible routes of administration that will produce the desired therapeutic effect (e.g., oral or topical), (3) patient characteristics (e.g., age, level of consciousness, ability to swallow a solid dosage form), (4)

specific characteristics of the disease being treated, (5) comfort for the patient, and (6) ease or convenience of administration.

In checking the physical form of each ingredient, the pharmacist should not confuse drug substances that are available in more than one form. For example, coal tar is available as Coal Tar, USP, or Coal Tar Topical Solution, USP; phenol is available as Liquified Phenol, USP, or Phenol, USP; sulfur is available as Precipitated Sulfur, USP, or Sublimed Sulfur, USP. If ingredi-ents are liquids, the pharmacist should consider compounding liquid dosage forms such as solutions, syrups, or elixirs for the final product. If ingredients are crystals or powders and the final dosage form is intended to be a dry dosage form, options such as divided powders (powder papers) or capsules should be considered. If ingredients are both liquids and dry forms, liquid formulations such as solutions, suspensions, elixirs, syrups, and emulsions should be considered.

Care must be exercised when using commercial drug products as a source of active ingredients. For example, extended-release or delayed-release products should not be crushed. Also, since chemicals such as preservatives and excipients in commercial products may affect the overall stability and bioavailability of the com-pounded product, their presence should not be ignored. Information on preservatives and excipients in specific commercial products can be found in package inserts and also in the dosage form section of selected product monographs in *USP DI Volume I.*[6]

If an injectable drug product is a possible source of active ingredient, the pharmacist should check the salt form of the injectable product to make sure it is the same salt form ordered. If it is necessary to use a different salt because of physical or chemical compatibility considerations or product availability, the pharmacist should consult with the prescriber. Some injectable products contain active constituents in the form of prodrugs that may not be active when adminis-tered by other routes. For example, if an injectable solution is a possible source of active ingredient for an oral product, the pharmacist must consider the stability of the drug in gastric fluids, the first-pass effect, and palatability. Also, if injectable powders for reconstitution are used, expiration dating may have to be quite short.

Storage

All chemicals and drug products must be stored according to *USP–NF* and manufacturer specifications. Most chemicals and drug products marketed for compounding use are packaged by the manufacturer in tight, light-resistant containers. Chemicals intended for compounding should be purchased in small quantities and stored in the manufacturer's original container, which is labeled with product and storage information. This Practice fosters the use of fresh chemicals and ensures that the manufacturer's label remains with the lot of chemical on hand. Certificates of purity for chemical ingredients should be filed for a period of time no less than the state's time requirement for retention of dispensing records.

The manufacturer's label instructions for storage should be followed explicitly to ensure the integrity of chemicals and drug products and to protect employees. Most chemicals and commercial drug products may be stored at controlled room temperature, between 15 and 30 °C (59 and 86 °F); however, the pharmacist should always check the manufacturer's label for any special storage requirements. Storage information provided for specific commercial drug products in *USP DI Volume I* and on product labels follows the definitions for storage temperatures found in the General Notices and Requirements section of *USP–NF*. An acceptable refrigerator maintains temperatures between 2 and 8 °C (36 and 46 °F); an acceptable freezer maintains temperatures between "20 and "10°C (" 4 to +14 °F)

To protect pharmacy employees and property, hazardous products such as acetone and flexible collodion must be stored appropriately. Safety storage cabinets in various sizes are available from laboratory suppliers.

Personnel

Compounding personnel include pharmacists and supportive personnel engaged in any aspect of the compounding procedures.

Training. The pharmacist—who is responsible for ensuring that the best technical knowledge and skill, most careful and accurate procedures, and prudent professional judgment are consistently applied in the compounding of pharmaceuticals—must supervise all compounding activities and ensure that supportive personnel are adequately trained to perform assigned functions. Both pharmacists and the compounding personnel they supervise should participate in programs designed to enhance and maintain competence in compounding. Training programs should include instruction in the following areas:

- Proper use of compounding equipment such as balances and measuring devices—

including guidelines for selecting proper measuring devices, limitations of weighing equipment and measuring apparatus, and the importance of accuracy in measuring.

- Pharmaceutical techniques needed for preparing compounded dosage forms (e.g., levigation, trituration, methods to increase dissolution, geometric dilution).

- Properties of dosage forms (see Pharmaceutical Dosage Forms in *USP–NF*) to be compounded and related factors such as stability, storage considerations, and handling procedures.

- Literature in which information on stability, solubility, and related material can be found (see suggested references at the end of this document).

- Handling of nonhazardous and hazardous materials in the work area, including protective measures for avoiding exposure, emergency procedures to follow in the event of exposure, and the location of Material Safety Data Sheets (MSDSs) in the facility.[7–10]

- Use and interpretation of chemical and pharmaceutical symbols and abbreviations in medication orders and in product formulation directions.

- Pharmaceutical calculations.

Procedures should be established to verify the ability of staff to meet established competencies. These procedures may include observation, written tests, or quality control testing of finished products.

Attire. Personnel engaged in compounding should wear clean clothing appropriate for the duties they perform. Protective apparel, such as head, face hand, and arm coverings, should be worn as necessary to preclude contamination of products and to protect workers.

Generally, a clean laboratory jacket is considered appropriate attire for most personnel performing nonsterile compounding activities. Personnel involved in compounding hazardous materials should wear safety goggles, gloves, a mask or respirator, double gowns, and foot covers as required, depending on the substance being handled. To avoid microbial contamination of compounded drug products, written policies should be established that address appropriate precautions to be observed if an employee has an open lesion or an illness. Depending on the situation, an affected employee may be required to wear special protective apparel, such as a mask or gloves, or may be directed to avoid all contact with compounding procedures.

Reference Materials

Pharmacists and supportive personnel must have ready access to reference materials on all aspects of compounding (see suggested references at the end of this document). Earlier editions of some references, such as *Remington's Pharmaceutical Sciences,* provide more comprehensive compounding information than do the later editions. Information on compounding extemporaneous dosage forms from commercially available products can sometimes be obtained from the product's FDA-approved labeling (package insert), the manufacturer, a local pharmacy college, or a drug information center. It is essential that the stability and proper storage conditions for extemporaneous products be thoroughly researched. Therefore, the availability of adequate references and appropriate training in the use of the references is important.

Documentation and Record Keeping

Each step of the compounding process should be documented. Pharmacists should maintain at least four sets of records in the compounding area: (1) compounding formulas and procedures, (2) a log of all compounded items, including batch records and sample batch labels (see section on packaging and labeling), (3) equipment-maintenance records, including documentation of checks of balances, refrigerators, and freezers, and (4) a record of ingredients purchased, including certificates of purity for chemicals (see section on ingredient selection) and MSDSs.

Compounding procedures should be documented in enough detail that preparations can be replicated and the history of each ingredient can be traced. Documentation should include a record of who prepared the product (if the compounder is not a pharmacist, the supervising pharmacist should also sign the compounding record); all names, lot numbers, and quantities of ingredients used; the order of mixing, including any interim procedures used (such as preparing a solution and using an aliquot); the assigned beyond-use date; and any special storage requirements (see section on stability and expiration dating). Compounding formulas and procedures should be written in a typeface that can be read easily. If formulas originate from published articles, copies of the articles should be attached to or filed with the written procedures.

Equipment maintenance and calibrations should be documented and the record maintained in an equipment-maintenance record file.

Refrigerator and freezer thermometers should be checked and documented routinely, as should alarm systems indicating that temperatures are outside of acceptable limits.

Follow-up contact with patients who have received extemporaneously compounded products is recommended to ascertain that the product is physically stable and that no adverse effects have occurred from use of the product. Documentation of the contact and the findings is recommended.

Stability, Expiration, and Beyond-Use Dating

The *USP–NF*[4] defines stability as the extent to which a dosage form retains, within specified limits and throughout its period of storage and use, the same properties and characteristics that it possessed at the time of its preparation. The *USP–NF* lists the following five types of stability:

- Chemical
- Physical
- Microbiological
- Therapeutic
- Toxicological

Factors affecting stability include the properties of each ingredient, whether therapeutically active or inactive. Environmental factors such as temperature, radiation, light, humidity, and air can also affect stability. Similarly, such factors as particle size, pH, the properties of water and other solvents employed, the nature of the container, and the presence of other substances resulting from contamination or from the intentional mixing of products can influence stability.[4]

Since compounded drug products are intended for consumption immediately or storage for a very limited time, stability evaluation and expiration dating are different for these products than for manufactured drug products. According to criteria for assigning dating in the *USP–NF*[4] General Notices and Requirements section and the Code of Federal Regulations,[11] the pharmacist labeling extemporaneously compounded drug products should be concerned with the beyond-use date as used by *USP–NF* or the expiration date as used by the Code of Federal Regulations. For uniformity, the term *beyond-use date* will be used in the remainder of this bulletin. The beyond-use date is defined as that date after which a dispensed product should no longer be used by a patient.

Determination of the period during which a compounded product may be usable after dispensing should be based on available stability information and reasonable patient needs with respect to the intended drug therapy. When a commercial drug product is used as a source of active ingredient, its expiration date can often be used as a factor in determining a beyond-use date. For stability or expiration information on commercial drug products, the pharmacist can refer to *USP DI Volume I*.[6] If no information is available, the manufacturer should be contacted. When the active ingredient is a USP or NF product, the pharmacist may be able to use the expiration dating of similar commercial products for guidance in assigning a beyond-use date. In addition, the pharmacist can often refer to published literature to obtain stability data on the same active ingredient under varying conditions and in different formulations.[12]

The pharmacist must assess the potential for instability that may result from the new environment for the active ingredients—from the combination of ingredients and the packaging materials. According to *USP–NF*,[4] hydrolysis, oxidation-reduction, and photolysis are the most common chemical reactions that cause instability. When the possibility of such reactions exists, the pharmacist should seek additional stability data or consider other approaches. These could, in extreme cases, include the preparation and dispensing of more than one compounded drug product or the use of alternative methods of dosing. For some drugs, the latter methods might include, for example, crushing a tablet or emptying the contents of a hard gelatin capsule into an appropriate food substance at each dosing time.

In assigning a beyond-use date for compounded drug products, the pharmacist should use all available stability information, plus education and experience in deciding how factors affecting product stability should be weighted. In the absence of stability data to the contrary or any indication of a stability problem, the following general criteria for assigning maximum beyond-use dates are recommended. It must be emphasized that these are *general* criteria. Professional judgment as discussed elsewhere in this section must be used in deciding when these general criteria may not be appropriate.

- When a manufactured final-dosage-form product is used as a source of active ingredient, use no more than 25% of the manufacturer's remaining expiration dating or six months, whichever is less;

- When a USP or NF chemical not from a manufactured final-dosage-form product is used, use no more than six months;

- In other cases, use the intended period of therapy or no more than 30 days, whichever is less.

All compounded products should be observed for signs of instability. Observations should be performed during preparation of the drug product and any storage period that may occur before the compounded drug product is dispensed. A list of observable indications of instability for solid, liquid, and semisolid dosage forms appears in *USP–NF*.

Packaging and Labeling

The packaging of extemporaneously compounded products for ambulatory patients should comply with regulations pertaining to the Poison Prevention Packaging Act of 1970. These regulations can be found in *USP–NF*.[4]

Containers for compounded products should be appropriate for the dosage form compounded. For example, to minimize administration errors, oral liquids should never be packaged in syringes intended to be used for injection.

The drug product container should not interact physically or chemically with the product so as to alter the strength, quality, or purity of the compounded product. Glass and plastic are commonly used in containers for compounded products. To ensure container inertness, visibility, strength, rigidity, moisture protection, ease of reclosure, and economy of packaging, glass containers have been the most widely used for compounded products.[3] Amber glass and some plastic containers may be used to protect light-sensitive products from degradation; however, glass that transmits ultraviolet or violet light rays (this includes green, blue, and clear ["flint"] glass) should not be used to protect light-sensitive products.

The use of plastic containers for compounded products has increased because plastic is less expensive and lighter in weight than glass. Since compounded products are intended for immediate use, most capsules, ointments, and creams should be stable in high-density plastic vials or ointment jars. Only plastic containers meeting *USP–NF* standards should be used.[4] Reclosable plastic bags may be acceptable for selected divided powders that are intended to be used within a short period of time.

Each compounded product should be appropriately labeled according to state and federal regulations. Labels should include the generic or chemical name of active ingredients, strength or quantity, pharmacy lot number, beyond-use date, and any special storage requirements. If a commercial product has been used as a source of drug, the generic name of the product should be used on the label. The trade name should not be used because, once the commercial drug product has been altered, it no longer exists as the approved commercial product. Listing the names and quantities of inactive ingredients on labels is also encouraged. The coining of short names for convenience (e.g., "Johnson's solution") is strongly discouraged; these names provide no assistance to others who may need to identify ingredients (e.g., in emergency circumstances).

Capsules should be labeled with the quantity (micrograms or milligrams) of active ingredient(s) per capsule. Oral liquids should be labeled with the strength or concentration per dose (e.g., 125 mg/5 mL or 10 meq/15 mL). If the quantity of an active ingredient is a whole number, the number should not be typed with a decimal point followed by a zero. For example, the strength of a capsule containing 25 mg of active ingredient should be labeled as 25 mg and not 25.0 mg. In cases where the dosage strength is less than a whole number, a zero should precede the decimal point (e.g., 0.25 µg).[3]

In expressing salt forms of chemicals on a label, it is permissible to use atomic abbreviations. For example, HCl may be used for hydrochloride, HBr for hydrobromide, Na for sodium, and K for potassium.

Vehicles should also be stated on labels, especially if similar products are prepared with different vehicles. For example, if a pharmacist prepares two potassium syrups, one using Syrup, USP, as the vehicle and one using a sugar-free syrup as the vehicle, the name of the vehicle should be included on the labels.

Liquids and semisolid concentrations may be expressed in terms of percentages. When the term "percent" or the symbol "%" is used without qualification for solids and semisolids, percent refers to weight in weight; for solutions or suspensions, percent refers to weight in volume; for solutions of liquids in liquids, percent refers to volume in volume.[4]

Labels for compounded products that are prepared in batches should include a pharmacy-assigned lot number. Assignment of a pharmacy lot number must enable the history of the compounded product to be traced, including the person compounding the product and the product's formula, ingredients, and procedures. Being able to trace the history of a batch is essential in cases of a drug product recall or withdrawal.

In the preparation of labels for batches of compounded products, all extra labels should be destroyed, since pharmacy lot numbers change with each batch. If computers, memory typewriters, or label machines are used to print batch labels, care must be taken to ensure that the memory and printing mechanism have been cleared and the correct information is programmed before any additional labels are made. It is a good practice to run a blank label between each batch of labels to ensure that the memory has been erased or cleared. To document the information printed on each set of labels, a sample label printed for the batch should be attached to the compounded-product log. If labels are sequentially prepared for different drug products, procedures should exist to minimize the risk of mislabeling the compounded products. These procedures should ensure, for example, that labels for one drug product are physically well separated from labels for any other drug product.

Auxiliary labels are convenient for conveying special storage or use information. Auxiliary labels should be attached conspicuously to containers, if possible. If the container is too small for both a general label and an auxiliary label, special storage and use instructions should appear on the label in a format that will emphasize the instructions.

Limited Batch Compounding

The purpose of extemporaneously compounding products is to provide individualized drug therapy for a particular patient. When a pharmacist is repeatedly asked to prepare identical compounded products, it may be reasonable and more efficient for the pharmacist to prepare small batches of the compounded product.

Batch sizes should be consistent with the volume of drug orders or prescriptions the pharmacist receives for the compounded product and the stability of the compounded product. The pharmacist should use judgment in deciding reasonable batch sizes. Product assays should be performed by a chemical analysis laboratory on a regular basis to ensure product consistency among various lots, product uniformity, and stability. Analyses should be repeated every time an ingredient (active or inert) or procedure is changed. Documentation of assay findings should be filed for a period no less than the state's time requirement for the retention of dispensing records.

General Compounding Considerations

To provide the patient with the most stable drug product, the pharmacist should take the following steps upon receiving a prescription order that requires compounding.

First, the pharmacist should determine if a similar commercial product is available. A pharmacist can refer to various reference texts to check the availability of identical or similar products. Package inserts from commercially available products also contain information on inactive ingredients that can be compared with the requested formulation. If there is a commercially manufactured identical product, the local availability of the product should be determined.

When a similar product is commercially available, the pharmacist should determine which ingredients are different from the requested formulation to decide whether or not the commercial product can be used. At this stage, the pharmacist should seek answers to the following questions:

- Are all of the ingredients appropriate for the condition being treated?

- Are the concentrations of the ingredients in the drug order reasonable?

- Are the physical, chemical, and therapeutic properties of the individual ingredients consistent with the expected properties of the ordered drug product?

If the answers to these questions are positive, the pharmacist should consult the prescriber about the possibility of dispensing the commercial product. (In some states, pharmacists may not be required to obtain permission from the prescriber to dispense a commercial product if the formulation is identical to the drug order.) Dispensing a commercial product is preferable to extemporaneously compounding a drug product because commercial products carry the manufacturer's guarantee of labeled potency and stability.

If there is not a commercial product available with the same or similar formulation, the pharmacist should consider asking the prescriber the following questions:

- What is the purpose of the order? There may be another way to achieve the purpose without compounding a product.

- Where did the formula originate (article, meeting, colleague)?

- How will the drug product be used?

- Does the patient have other conditions that must be considered?

- For how long will the drug product be used?

If possible, the pharmacist should obtain a copy of the original formula to determine the extent to which the formulation has been tested for stability. When documentation is not available, the pharmacist should review the ingredients for appropriateness and reasonable concentrations.

For drug products that must be compounded, the pharmacist should closely observe the compounded drug product for any signs of instability. Such observations should be performed during preparation of the drug product and during any storage period that may occur before the compounded drug product is dispensed.

If specific packaging information is not available, a light-resistant, tight container, such as an amber vial or bottle, should be used to maximize stability (see section on packaging and labeling).

The pharmacist should label the compounded drug product, including an appropriate beyond-use date and storage instructions for the patient.

Specific Compounding Considerations

Accepted, proven compounding procedures for products including solutions, suspensions, creams, ointments, capsules, suppositories, troches, emulsions, and powders may be found in reference sources or the pharmacy literature. For additional information, pharmacists should check references cited in this document or consult colleagues or colleges of pharmacy with known expertise in compounding.

Glossary

For the purposes of this document, the following terms are used with the meanings shown.

Active Ingredient: Any chemical that is intended to furnish pharmacologic activity in the diagnosis, cure, mitigation, treatment, or prevention of disease or to affect the structure or function of the body of man or other animals.[4]

Batch: Multiple containers of a drug product or other material with uniform character and quality, within specified limits, that are prepared in anticipation of prescription drug orders based on routine, regularly observed prescribing patterns.

Cold: Any temperature not exceeding 8 °C (46 °F).[4]

Commercially Available Product: Any drug product manufactured by a producer registered with the Department of Health and Human Services as a pharmaceutical manufacturer.

Compounding: The mixing of substances to prepare a drug product.

Container: A device that holds a drug product and is or may be in direct contact with the product.[3]

Cool: Any temperature between 8 and 15 °C (46 and 59 °F).[4]

Drug Product: A finished dosage form that contains an active drug ingredient usually, but not necessarily (in the case of a placebo), in combination with inactive ingredients.[4]

Extemporaneous: Impromptu; prepared without a standard formula from an official compendium; prepared as required for a specific patient.

Inactive Ingredient: Any chemical other than the active ingredients in a drug product.[4]

Manufacturer: Anyone registered with the Department of Health and Human Services as a producer of drug products.[14]

Sensitivity Requirements: The maximal load that will cause one subdivision of change on the index plate in the position of rest of the indicator of the balance.[4]

Stability: The chemical and physical integrity of a drug product over time.[4]

Trituration: The reducing of substances to fine particles by rubbing them in a mortar with a pestle.[3]

Warm: Any temperature between 30 and 40 °C (86 and 104 °F).[4]

Suggested References

Product Availability

American Drug Index

Drug Facts & Comparisons

Physicians' Desk Reference

The Extra Pharmacopoeia (Martindale)

CHEMSOURCES

AHFS Drug Information

Compounding Techniques

Compounding Companion PC-Based Software

King's *Dispensing of Medications*

Remington's *Pharmaceutical Sciences*

Contemporary Compounding column in *U.S. Pharmacist*

Pharmaceutical Calculations

Stoklosa and Ansel's *Pharmaceutical Calculations*

Math—Use It or Lose It column in *Hospital Pharmacy*

Calculations in Pharmacy column in *U.S. Pharmacist*

Drug Stability and Compatibility

American Journal of Hospital Pharmacy

ASHP's *Handbook on Extemporaneous Formulations*

ASHP's *Handbook on Injectable Drugs*

International Pharmaceutical Abstracts

Journal of the Parenteral Drug Association (now *Journal of Pharmaceutical Science and Technology*)

Canadian Society of Hospital Pharmacists *Extemporaneous Oral Liquid Dosage Preparations*

Pediatric Drug Formulations

Physicians' Desk Reference

Contemporary Compounding column in *U.S. Pharmacist*

AHFS Drug Information

The Merck Index

References

1. Pancorbo SA, Campagna KD, Devenport JK, et al. Task force report of competency statements for pharmacy practice. *Am J Pharm Educ.* 1987;51:196–206.

2. Allen LV Jr. Establishing and marketing your extemporaneous compounding service. *US Pharm.* 1990;15(Dec):74–7.

3. *Remington's Pharmaceutical Sciences.* 18th ed. Gennaro AR, ed. Easton, PA: Mack Publishing; 1990;1630–1, 1658, 1660.

4. *The United States Pharmacopeia*, 22nd rev., and *The National Formulary*, 17th ed. Rockville, MD: The United States Pharmacopeial Convention; 1989.

5. *USP DI Volume III: Approved Drug Products and Legal Requirements.* 14th ed. Rockville, MD: The United States Pharmacopeial Convention; 1994.

6. *USP DI Volume I: Drug Information for the Health Care Professional.* 14th ed. Rockville, MD: The United States Pharmacopeial Convention; 1994.

7. 29 §C.F.R. 1910. 1200(1990).

8. ASHP technical assistance bulletin on handling cytotoxic and hazardous drugs. *Am J Hosp Pharm*. 1990;47:1033–49.

9. Feinberg JL. Complying with OSHA's Hazard Communication Standard. *Consult Pharm*. 1991;6:444, 446, 448.

10. Myers CE. Applicability of OSHA Hazard Communication Standard to drug products. *Am J Hosp Pharm*. 1990;47:1960–1.

11. 21 C.F.R. §211.137.

12. Connors KA, Amidon GL, Stella VJ. *Chemical Stability of Pharmaceuticals: A Handbook for Pharmacists*. 2nd ed. New York: Wiley; 1986.

13. American Society of Hospital Pharmacists. ASHP guidelines on preventing medication errors in hospitals. *Am J Hosp Pharm*. 1993; 50:305–14.

14. Fitzgerald WL Jr. The legal authority to compound in pharmacy practice. *Tenn Pharm*. 1990;26(Mar):21–2.

Approved by the ASHP Board of Directors, April 27, 1994. Developed by the Council on Professional Affairs.

The bibliographic citation for this document is as follows: American Society of Hospital Pharmacists. ASHP technical assistance bulletin on compounding nonsterile products in pharmacies. *Am J Hosp Pharm*. 1994; 51:1441–8.

ASHP Guidelines on Pharmacy-Prepared Ophthalmic Products

Pharmacists are frequently called on to prepare sterile products intended for ophthalmic administration when a suitable sterile ophthalmic product is not available from a licensed manufacturer. These products may be administered topically or by subconjunctival or intraocular (e.g., intravitreal and intracameral) injection and may be in the form of solutions, suspensions, or ointments.

The sterility of these products, as well as accuracy in the calculation and preparation of doses, is of great importance. Ocular infections and loss of vision caused by contamination of extemporaneously prepared ophthalmic products have been reported.[1,2] Drugs administered by subconjunctival or intraocular injection often have narrow therapeutic indices. In practice, serious errors in technique have occurred in the preparation of intravitreal solutions, which resulted in concentrations up to double the intended amounts.[3] To ensure adequate stability, uniformity, and sterility, ophthalmic products from licensed manufacturers should be used whenever possible.

The following guidelines are intended to assist pharmacists when extemporaneous preparation of ophthalmic products is necessary. These guidelines do not apply to the manufacturing of sterile pharmaceuticals as defined in state and federal laws and regulations. Other guidelines on extemporaneous compounding of ophthalmic products also have been published.[4,5]

1. Before compounding any product for ophthalmic use, the pharmacist should review documentation that substantiates the safety and benefit of the product when administered into the eye. If no such documentation is available, the pharmacist must employ professional judgment in determining suitability of the product for ophthalmic administration.

2. Important factors to be considered in preparing an ophthalmic medication include the following:[6]

    a. Sterility.

    b. Tonicity.

    c. pH, buffering.

    d. Inherent toxicity of the drug.

    e. Need for a preservative.

    f. Solubility.

    g. Stability in an appropriate vehicle.

    h. Viscosity.

    i. Packaging and storage of the finished product.

3. A written procedure for each ophthalmic product compounded should be established and kept on file and should be easily retrievable. The procedure should specify appropriate steps in compounding, including aseptic methods, and whether microbiologic filtration or terminal sterilization (e.g., autoclaving) of the finished product is appropriate.

4. Before preparation of the product is begun, mathematical calculations should be reviewed by another person or by an alternative method of calculation in order to minimize error. This approach is especially important for products, such as intraocular injections, for which extremely small doses are frequently ordered, necessitating multiple dilutions. Decimal errors in the preparation of these products may have serious consequences.

5. Accuracy in compounding ophthalmic products is further enhanced by the use of larger volumes, which tends to diminish the effect of errors in measurement caused by the inherent inaccuracy of measuring devices. Larger volumes, however, also necessitate special attention to adequate mixing procedures, especially for ointments.

6. Strict adherence to aseptic technique and proper sterilization procedures are crucial in the preparation of ophthalmic products. All extemporaneous compounding of ophthalmic products should be performed in a certified laminar airflow hood (or, for preparing cytotoxic or hazardous agents, a biological safety cabinet).[5] Only personnel trained and proficient in the techniques and procedures should prepare ophthalmic products. Quality-assurance principles for compounding sterile products should be followed, and methods should be established to validate all procedures and processes related to sterile product preparation. In addition, the following should be considered:

a. Ingredients should be mixed in sterile empty containers. Individual ingredients often can first be drawn into separate syringes and then injected into a larger syringe by insertion of the needles into the needle-free tip of the larger syringe. The larger syringe should be of sufficient size to allow for proper mixing of ingredients.

b. To maximize measurement accuracy, the smallest syringe appropriate for measuring the required volume should be used. When the use of a single syringe would require estimation of the volume (e.g., measuring 4.5 ml in a 5-ml syringe with no mark at the 4.5-ml level), the use of two syringes of appropriate capacities (or two separate syringe "loads") should be considered in order to provide a more accurate measurement.

c. A fresh disposable needle and syringe should be used at each step to avoid contamination and prevent error due to residual contents.

d. When multiple dilutions are required, the containers of interim concentrations should be labeled to avoid confusion.

e. In the preparation of an ophthalmic product from either (1) a sterile powder that has been reconstituted or (2) a liquid from a glass ampul, the ingredients should be filtered through a 5-μm filter to remove any particulate matter.

7. For ophthalmic preparations that must be sterilized, an appropriate and validated method of sterilization should be determined on the basis of the characteristics of the particular product and container. Filtration of the preparation through a 0.22-μm filter into a sterile final container is a commonly used method; however, this method is not suitable for sterilizing ophthalmic suspensions and ointments.[7] When an ophthalmic preparation is compounded from a nonsterile ingredient, the final product must be sterilized before it is dispensed. Sterilization by autoclaving in the final container may be possible, provided that product stability is not adversely affected and appropriate quality control procedures are followed.[6]

8. Preservative-free ingredients should be used in the preparation of intraocular injections, since some preservatives are known to be toxic to many of the internal structures of the eye.[6]

9. In the preparation of ophthalmic products from cytotoxic or other hazardous agents, the pharmacist should adhere to established safety guidelines for handling such agents.[8,9]

10. The final container should be appropriate for the ophthalmic product and its intended use and should not interfere with the stability and efficacy of the preparation.[10] Many ophthalmic liquids can be packaged in sterile plastic bottles with self-contained dropper tips or in glass bottles with separate droppers. Ophthalmic ointments should be packaged in sterilized ophthalmic tubes. Injectables that are not for immediate use should be packaged in sterile vials rather than in syringes, and appropriate overfill should be included. All containers should be adequately sealed to prevent contamination.

11. The pharmacist should assign appropriate expiration dates to extemporaneously prepared ophthalmic products; these dates should be based on documented stability data as well as the potential for microbial contamination of the product.[11] The chemical stability of the active ingredient, the preservative, and packaging material should be considered in determining the over-all stability of the final ophthalmic product.[12]

12. Ophthalmic products should be clearly and accurately labeled. In some cases, it may be appropriate to label the products with both the weight and concentration of active ingredients and preservatives. Labels should also specify storage and handling requirements and expiration dates. Extemporaneously prepared ophthalmic products dispensed for outpatient use should be labeled in accordance with applicable state regulations for prescription labeling.

References

1. Associated Press. Pittsburgh woman loses eye to tainted drugs; 12 hurt. *Baltimore Sun.* 1990;Nov 9:3A.

2. Associated Press. Eye drop injuries prompt an FDA warning. *N Y Times.* 1990;140(Dec 9):391.

3. Jeglum EL, Rosenberg SB, Benson WE. Preparation of intravitreal drug doses. *Ophthalmic Surg.* 1981;12:355–9.

4. Reynolds LA. Guidelines for preparation of sterile ophthalmic products. *Am J Hosp Pharm.* 1991;48:2438–9.

5. Reynolds LA, Closson R. *Ophthalmic Drug Formulations. A Handbook of Extemporaneous Products.* Vancouver, WA: Applied Therapeutics; (in press).

6. *The United States Pharmacopeia*, 22nd rev., and *The National Formulary*, 17th ed. Rockville, MD: The United States Pharmacopeial Convention; 1989:1692–3.

7. Allen LV. Indomethacin 1% ophthalmic suspension. *US Pharm.* 1991;16(May):82–3.

8. American Society of Hospital Pharmacists. ASHP technical assistance bulletin on handling cytotoxic and hazardous drugs. *Am J Hosp Pharm.* 1990;47:1033–49.

9. OSHA work-practice guidelines for personnel dealing with cytotoxic (antineoplastic) drugs. *Am J Hosp Pharm.* 1986;43:1193–204.

10. Ansel HC, Popovich NG. *Pharmaceutical Dosage Forms and Drug Delivery Systems.* 5th ed. Philadelphia: Lea & Febiger; 1990:354–7.

11. Stolar MH. Expiration dates of repackaged drug products. *Am J Hosp Pharm.* 1979; 36:170. Editorial.

12. *Remington's Pharmaceutical Sciences.* 19th ed. Gennaro AR, ed. Easton, PA: Mack Publishing; 1990:1581–959.

These guidelines were reviewed in 2008 by the Council on Pharmacy Practice and by the Board of Directors and were found to still be appropriate.

Approved by the ASHP Board of Directors, April 21, 1993. Developed by the ASHP Council on Professional Affairs.

The bibliographic citation for this document is as follows: American Society of Hospital Pharmacists. ASHP technical assistance bulletin on pharmacy-prepared ophthalmic products. *Am J Hosp Pharm.* 1993; 50:1462–3. Table 1.